Presented to

By Lederle Laboratories
Makers of Lederfen and Lederspan
As a service to medicine

Lederle

Lederle Laboratories, a division of Cyanamid of Great Britain Limited,
Fareham Road, Gosport, Hants. PO13 0AS. Tel: (0329) 224000.

RHEUMATOLOGY

MANAGEMENT OF COMMON DISEASES IN FAMILY PRACTICE

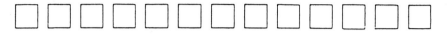

Series Editors: J. Fry and M. Lancaster-Smith

RHEUMATOLOGY

H. Berry, MA DM FRCP

Consultant Physician, Department of Rheumatology and Rehabilitation, Kings College Hospital, London

and

A. S. M. Jawad, DMedRehab DCH MRCP

Senior Registrar, Department of Rheumatology and Rehabilitation, Kings College Hospital, London

MTP PRESS LIMITED
a member of the KLUWER ACADEMIC PUBLISHERS GROUP
LANCASTER / BOSTON / THE HAGUE / DORDRECHT

G

Published in the UK and Europe by
MTP Press Limited
Falcon House
Lancaster, England

British Library Cataloguing in Publication Data

Berry, H.
   Rheumatology. – (Management of common diseases in family practice)
   1. Rheumatism
   I. Title   II. Jawad, A.S.M.   III. Series
   616.7'23   RC927

ISBN 0-85200-900-3
ISBN 0-85200-794-9 series

Published in the USA by
MTP Press Limited
A division of Kluwer Boston Inc.
190 Old Derby Street
Hingham, MA 02043, USA

Typeset by UPS Blackburn Limited, 76-80 Northgate, Blackburn, Lancashire BB2 1AB.
Printed by Butler and Tanner Ltd, Frome and London.

_ 5MAY1995

Contents

v

Series Editor's Foreword

□ □ □ □ □ □ □ □ □ □ □ □

Effective management logically follows accurate diagnosis. Such logic often is difficult to apply in practice. Absolute diagnostic accuracy may not be possible, particularly in the field of primary care, when management has to be on analysis of symptoms and on knowledge of the individual patient and family.

This series follows that on *Problems in Practice* which was concerned more with diagnosis in the widest sense and this series deals more definitively with general care and specific treatment of symptoms and diseases.

Good management must include knowledge of the nature, course and outcome of the conditions, as well as prominent clinical features and assessment and investigations, but the emphasis is on what to do best for the patient.

Family medical practitioners have particular difficulties and advantages in their work. Because they often work in professional isolation in the community and deal with relatively small numbers of near-normal patients their experience with the more serious and more rare conditions is restricted. They find it difficult to remain up-to-date with medical advances and even more difficult to decide on the suitability and application of new and relatively untried methods compared with those that are 'old' and well proven.

Their advantages are that because of long-term continuous care for their patients they have come to know them and their families well and are able to become familiar with the more common and less serious diseases of their communities.

This series aims to correct these disadvantages by providing practical information and advice on the less common, potentially serious conditions, but at the same time to take note of the special features of general medical practice.

To achieve these objectives, the *titles* are intentionally those of accepted body systems and population groups.

The *experience bases* are those of the district general hospital and family practice. It is here that the day-to-day problems arise.

The *advice and presentation* are practical and have come from many years of conjoint experience of family and hospital practice.

The *series* is intended for family practitioners – the young and the less than young. All should benefit and profit from comparing the views of the authors with their own. Many will coincide, some will be accepted as new, useful and worthy of application and others may not be acceptable, but nevertheless will stimulate thought and enquiry.

Since medical care in the community and in hospitals involves teamwork, this series also should be of relevance to nurses and others involved in personal and family care.

JOHN FRY
M. LANCASTER-SMITH

1

The Single Painful Swollen Joint

Table 1.1 *Common causes of the single painful joint*

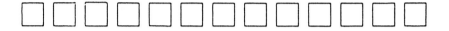

Trauma
Rheumatoid arthritis
Psoriatic arthritis
Reiter's syndrome
Osteoarthritis
Gout
Pseudogout
Infective arthritis
Systemic lupus erythematosus
Polyarteritis nodosa
Villonodular synovitis
Other rare causes

The presentation of a patient with a painful swollen joint is often an acute emergency causing the patient very considerable pain and discomfort. Unless a full history and a very careful examination is undertaken, the patient may suffer from an incorrect diagnosis and incorrect therapy. There are two immediate 'dont's':

(1) Do not give antibiotics without a positive bacteriological diagnosis.

(2) Do not put corticosteroids into the joint under any

circumstances unless you are sure that you have excluded infection.

This problem is one *par excellence* where a close relationship between the hospital outpatient department and the local general practitioner is essential. If there is any question as to the diagnosis, these patients should be sent to the hospital casualty department or rheumatology clinic for urgent consultation. An intra-articular aspiration and the use of the bacteriology or chemical pathology services may give an immediate diagnosis.

HISTORY

Sometimes the history will give an immediate answer, for example a patient with symmetrical polyarthritis elsewhere may suddenly have another joint involved which can indicate rheumatoid arthritis. The patient may give a history of trauma, for example a sporting or road traffic accident. There may be sexual exposure leading one to think of Reiter's syndrome or gonococcal arthritis. There may have been a previous history of skin disease such as psoriasis, bowel diseases such as ulcerative colitis or Crohn's disease, or a history of diarrhoea which could suggest the diagnosis of a reactive arthritis. One must not forget sacro-ilitis or ankylosing spondylitis. A history of previous attacks of pain in the big toe might indicate the presence of gout. The patient may have visited far-off countries which could indicate some underlying reaction by the joint to an existing infection: *Salmonella* or *Shigella* infection comes to mind.

There may have been a history of recurrent attacks in the joint which could give rise to the possibility of pseudogout or villonodular synovitis. A recurring swollen knee is also found with a cartilage tear which can give considerable pain and discomfort; the history here may include the knee actually locking and buckling under the patient when he or she attempts to walk.

Table 1.2 *History*

Trauma and mechanical causes
Other joints
Sexual exposure
Skin disease e.g. psoriasis
Ankylosing spondylitis
Gout/pseudogout
Diarrhoea

EXAMINATION

A careful examination of the affected joint itself is clearly indicated. Look at the muscles above and below for wasting indicating chronicity of symptoms. The joint may be hot from almost all causes, but this does not necessarily indicate infection. In the knee, tenderness over the joint margin medially may indicate a medial meniscal tear. A search elsewhere may reveal psoriatic plaques or symmetrical polyarthritis or rheumatoid nodules. One should also check for a urethral discharge, a careful look at the eyes for evidence of uveitis is sometimes helpful, and a check for balanitis may be indicated.

Table 1.3 *Examination*

Muscle wasting
Joint tenderness
Skin plaques or nodules
Urethral discharge
Eyes

ACTION

If the diagnosis is still in doubt, the next investigation is to aspirate the joint. The aspirate should be observed to see whether it is turbid or clear. Turbidity indicates the presence of large numbers of cells which may be polymorphonuclear as well as lymphocytes. The presence of a high count indicates inflammation which may have arisen as a result of an infection or an inflammatory joint. Counts of 40 000 to 50 000 white cells per cubic millimetre are found not only in infection but also in rheumatoid and psoriatic disease. A search for organisms is important: Gram stain is used to look for intracellular diplococci to exclude gonococcal infection, and clumps of cocci to exclude staphylococci or chains of streptococci. A Ziehl–Neelsen stain is also indicated to exclude the unusual presence of mycobacterium tuberculosis in a joint. The reactive arthropathies give a high fluid count with few cells, and osteoarthritic knee effusions rarely have white cell counts in excess of 1 000 per cubic millimetre. It is rare to find organisms of *Salmonella* and *Shigella* in the joints due to a reactive cause. Syphilis can occasionally cause an acute joint reaction, either due to an infective joint (in which case dark ground illumination will reveal the spirochaete), or to a reactive arthritis which will not reveal organisms.

A search for crystals is carried out using a polarizing microscope. Strongly negative birefringence indicates gout (urate crystals), whereas weakly positive birefringence indicates pseudogout (pyrophosphate crystals). Hydroxyapatite is now accepted as a cause of low-grade joint inflammation, but spectrophotometry is required in order to isolate the crystals.

Laboratory tests

The white cell count may be elevated in infection and the haemoglobin may be reduced in chronic inflammatory disease. The ESR will inevitably be raised in the presence of an active disease. The latex may be positive in the presence of rheumatoid arthritis, but negative for osteoarthritis. The antinuclear factor (ANF) will be positive along with the DNA binding for patients with systemic lupus erythematosus. Polyarthritis nodosa is best diagnosed by the history of systemic disease involving gut and lungs, and by the exclusion of other causes as there is no specific diagnostic test. The

HBsAg antigen, 'Australia antigen,' may be positive in this condition in up to 20% of patients. The presence of a raised level of uric acid *on its own* does not indicate the presence of gout: it would, however, confirm a gouty tendency and if crystals are found this supports the diagnosis. There is no serum diagnostic test for pseudogout or apatite disease. The presence of skin psoriasis with a negative latex test is helpful in the diagnosis of psoriatic disease of the joints, 90% of these patients having pitting of the nails which is also a diagnostic aid.

Table 1.4 *Action: aspirate*

Look for organisms	in synovial
Look for crystals	fluid
Laboratory tests	
Do ESR/Hb, WBC and differential count	
Latex/ANF/DNA binding	
Uric acid	

MANAGEMENT

Somebody with an acutely painful joint should be hospitalized. If infection has been diagnosed an appropriate antibiotic should be started, the joint should be kept in a splint and the patient should be kept on complete bed rest. Soluble aspirin 4 g daily is extremely helpful for this condition.

Table 1.5 *Management*

Hospitalize
Aspirin
Splint
Aspiration
Arthroscopy
Arthrogram
Biopsy

An acute reactive joint should be managed in the same way, by aspirating to near dryness and treatment with rest, splinting and soluble aspirin. The acute gout or pseudogout joint is best treated by the use of a high dose of a non-steroidal anti-inflammatory drug such as indome·'iacin, starting with a 100 mg dose followed two hours later by a 50 mg dose if necessary. A rheumatoid joint should first be aspirated in order to make certain that an infective pathology is not missed. If the cause is rheumatoid, instilling the hydrocortisone may be extremely pain-relieving and systemically helpful. The same is true for the psoriatic joint or other causes of inflammatory joint disease. It may be necessary in the presence of a reactive arthritis to exclude underlying pathology such as *Salmonella* or *Shigella* disease along with the sexually acquired disease type of pathologies: these may involve the use of an appropriate antibiotic to the infective agent. Surgery may be indicated in the treatment of a cartilage tear, or of villonodular synovitis in terms of carrying out a synovectomy. In patients where there is doubt about the diagnosis, it may be necessary to carry out both arthroscopy and arthrography. An arthroscopy will reveal many cartilage problems or synovitis, and it is possible to carry out a synovial biopsy through the arthroscope. A more formal synovial biopsy may be carried out through an open biopsy, although pathological information obtained from this is not always helpful in that it will indicate only the presence or absence of inflammation rather than its exact cause. Other rare causes of arthritis have not been included in this chapter, but such diseases as Behçet's syndrome, familial Mediterranean fever and sickle-cell disease should be mentioned at this point along with bleeding disorders such as Factor VIII and Factor IX deficiency diseases. Finally, trauma should be excluded by the presence of a bloody effusion, which can be found in conjunction with the haematological disease. This is where the history is all important.

PROGNOSIS

Provided an accurate diagnosis is made and an early treatment carried out, the prognosis is excellent. However, if the diagnosis is delayed and if fixed flexion occurs early, it may well be impossible to overcome this although serial plastering can be helpful. This is a good example of where combined management between the patient's general practitioner and the hospital is so important.

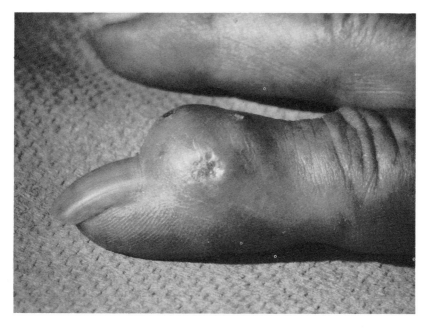

Figure 1.1   Acute gout in the terminal interphalangeal joint.

2

Polyarthralgia

By simple definition polyarthralgia means joint pain. It may appear in the presence of swelling which indicates polyarthritis (this is the subject of the following chapter). This chapter is devoted to how to approach a patient who comes into the clinic complaining only of joint pain without clinical evidence of any inflammation in the joint.

DIFFERENTIAL DIAGNOSIS

Polyarthralgia may be the presenting feature of rheumatoid arthritis, osteoarthritis, systemic lupus erythematosus and polyarteritis nodosa. It may rarely also be among the presenting features of all other arthropathies but these most commonly present with polyarthritis rather than polyarthralgia. There may, however, be a prodromal phase of these illnesses when the polyarthralgia is present and the inflammation has yet to develop.

HISTORY

As rheumatoid arthritis, osteoarthritis and the sero-negative arthropathies are discussed elsewhere, the emphasis in this chapter is

9

on systemic lupus erythematosus (SLE) and polyarteritis nodosa. A history of a skin rash, often with facial distribution across the bridge of the nose and possibly going on to the anterior chest wall, may be described by the patient suffering from systemic lupus erythematosus. The hair may also be affected, the patient describing a receding hair line and noticing that their hair is falling out leading to alopecia. The patient may complain of a cough or recurrent bouts of chest pain. Other complaints include shortness of breath, nocturia, polyarthralgia and neurological complications such as weakness of hand or foot, or recent onset of attacks of epilepsy.

A history of polyarthralgia accompanied by recurrent chest infection or recurrent attacks of diarrhoea along with a neurological complication suggests polyarteritis nodosa.

EXAMINATION

Examination of the patient suffering from possible SLE may reveal the 'butterfly' rash, as already described, across the bridge of the nose and even spreading to the anterior chest wall. This rash is different from that seen with discoid lupus erythematosus, where the rash tends not to cross the bridge of the nose and the lesions tend to be more circumscribed (hence the name). The relationship between discoid lupus and systemic lupus is unclear: some believe that discoid lupus is systemic lupus all along, the systemic complications developing later. In SLE it is common to find distorted hair follicles and a receding hair line along with alopecia. Lung findings include pleurisy, pleural effusion and pulmonary fibrosis. Cardiac involvement includes hypertension, pericarditis, cardiac murmurs and heart failure. All complications of this disease may be exacerbated by sitting in the sun. The hypertension is the result of renal disease and renal failure found in patients with this condition: it may be the presenting feature of the disease. Patients may become anuric if end-stage, with nausea. Vision may be disturbed because of the presence of papilloedema. Lupus can then lead to uveitis and Sjögren's syndrome with dry eyes and dry mouth. Arthralgia is

10

commonly seen, although arthritis is rare and deforming arthritis (Jaccoud's arthritis) is unusual in this condition.

With polyarteritis nodosa there may be few abnormal findings. There is no classic skin rash but occasionally patients have lung involvement with pleurisy, fibrosis and cor pulmonale. The heart may be involved with pericarditis; there may be (malignant phase) hypertension papilloedema, and an arthritis along with the arthralgia. Vasculitis with corkscrew lesions in the nail beds may be found.

INVESTIGATIONS

Investigations of the patient with SLE include full blood count, differential white count and ESR. The finding of a neutropenia is not uncommon; sometimes, however, these patients have a high white count. The haemoglobin is low as befits the anaemia of chronic disease. The ESR is often extremely high – over 100 mm per hour. The ANF is positive and sometimes strongly so; the rheumatoid factor may sometimes also be positive. The ANF tends to be more strongly positive than the rheumatoid factor in terms of titre. The confirmatory test here is the DNA binding which is positive in nearly all cases of patients with SLE. It is also positive in some patients where the ANF may be negative, these are patients who have unusual antinuclear antibodies such as anti-La or anti-Ro antibodies. Whether these patients have true lupus or whether they have mixed connective tissue disease with variant of lupus it is hard to be certain.

The investigation of polyarteritis nodosa is often much more difficult, and the diagnosis tends to be on the basis of excluding the other causes of polyarthralgia described above. 20% of patients have the finding of positive Australia antigen (HBsAg). A definitive investigation can be carried out using radiology, searching for aneurysmal dilatation of the renal arteriolar supply. This is a somewhat cumbersome investigation but may be necessary if there is no other way of being certain of the diagnosis. Muscle biopsy can reveal the presence of severe arteritic lesions with perivascular plugging and arteritic changes in the media and intima of the vessel wall.

TREATMENT

The management of a patient with SLE or polyarteritis nodosa is extremely difficult and often hazardous. The first advice for the patient suffering from systemic lupus is that they should probably keep out of the sun unless protected by a barrier cream, as the general condition can be exacerbated by the sun. The arthralgia and the arthritis should be treated with non-steroidal anti-inflammatory drugs. However, neurological complications, renal complications and possibly lung complications may well need corticosteroid therapy, prednisolone up to 40 mg or even 60 mg daily being necessary. High dosage is indicated particularly in the presence of the psychotic episodes which are a feature of this condition. Sometimes it is necessary to use immunosuppressive drugs which have the advantage of steroid sparing, this, however, means very careful monitoring in order to avoid the blood complications which are found with this therapy. Polyarteritis nodosa is also extremely difficult to treat. The use of corticosteroid therapy and immunosuppressive therapy is again indicated when life-threatening complications ensue.

Studies to evaluate whether or not patients with SLE should be treated with steroids and/or immunosuppressives have shown that the use of these agents does not in fact reduce either the death rate or the problems of the condition, the strong suggestion being that one should treat symptoms when they arise rather than trying therapy in any prophylactic way.

PROGNOSIS

Prognosis for SLE these days is very much better than it used to be. One suspects that this reflects better early diagnosis rather than overall improvement in management or a change in pattern of the disease. In the old days, these patients were only diagnosed when established renal or neurological complications had set in. However, 80% of patients are alive for at least 5 years in the latest UK series. The American series suggests that around 30% of those who present with renal or central nervous system complications will be alive at 8.4 years. With polyarteritis nodosa the figures are harder to elucidate, but again it would appear that providing patients are spared neurological and renal complications, the prognosis is reasonably good.

Table 2.1 *1982 revised criteria for classification of systemic lupus erythematosus**

Criterion		Definition
1. Malar rash		Fixed erythema, flat or raised, over the malar eminences, tending to spare the nasolabial folds
2. Discoid rash		Erythematous raised patches with adherent keratotic scaling and follicular plugging; atrophic scarring may occur in older lesions
3. Photosensitivity		Skin rash as a result of unusual reaction to sunlight, by patient history or physician observation
4. Oral ulcers		Oral or nasopharyngeal ulceration, usually painless, observed by a physician
5. Arthritis		Nonerosive arthritis involving 2 or more peripheral joints, characterized by tenderness, swelling or effusion
6. Serositis	a)	Pleuritis – convincing history of pleuritic pain or rub heard by a physician or evidence of pleural effusion *or*
	b)	Pericarditis – documented by ECG or rub or evidence of pericardial effusion
7. Renal disorder	a)	Persistent proteinuria greater than 0.5 grams per day or greater than 3 + if quantitation not performed *or*
	b)	Cellular casts – may be red cell, haemoglobin, granular, tubular, or mixed
8. Neurological disorder	a)	Seizures – in the absence of offending drugs or known metabolic derangements; e.g., uraemia, ketoacidosis, or electrolyte imbalance *or*
	b)	Psychosis – in the absence of offending drugs or known metabolic derangements, e.g., uraemia, ketoacidosis, or electrolyte imbalance

13

9. Haematological disorder	a)	Haemolytic anaemia – with reticulocytosis
		or
	b)	Leukopenia – less than 4000/mm³ total on 2 or more occasions
		or
	c)	Lymphopenia – less than 1500/mm³ on 2 or more occasions
		or
	d)	Thrombocytopenia – less than 100 000/mm³ in the absence of offending drugs
10. Immunological disorder	a)	Positive LE cell preparation
		or
	b)	Anti-DNA: antibody to native DNA in abnormal titre
		or
	c)	Anti-Sm: presence of antibody to Sm nuclear antigen
		or
	d)	False positive serological test for syphilis known to be positive for at least 6 months and confirmed by *Treponema pallidum* immobilization or fluorescent treponemal antibody absorption test
11. Antinuclear antibody		An abnormal titre of antinuclear antibody by immunofluorescence or an equivalent assay at any point in time and in the absence of drugs known to be associated with 'drug-induced lupus' syndrome

---

* The proposed classification is based on 11 criteria. For the purpose of identifying patients in clinical studies, a person shall be said to have systemic lupus erythematosus if any 4 or more of the 11 criteria are present, serially or simultaneously, during any interval of observation.

(From Tan, EM, Cohen, AS, Fries, JF, *et al.* (1982). The 1982 revised criteria for the classification of systemic lupus erythematosus *Arthritis Rheum.* **25,** 1271)

3

Polyarthritis

□ □ □ □ □ □ □ □ □ □ □ □ □ □

Polyarthritis presents a diagnostic and therapeutic challenge with many pitfalls for the unwary. One common fault is to assume automatically that polyarthritis must be rheumatoid arthritis, but there are many other causes of symmetrical polyarthritis which have to be excluded before this diagnosis is reached.

HISTORY

History here is all important. Did the swollen joints present together or separately? Was the onset sudden or gradual? Is the pattern consistent? A history of flitting arthritis may indicate rheumatoid arthritis with the palindromic onset. Asymmetrical joint pattern, particularly involving one terminal interphalangeal joint, may indicate psoriatic arthropathy. The presence of knee arthritis may indicate sarcoid or ankylosing spondylitis. Involvement of small joints of the feet may indicate the arthritis of either ulcerative colitis, Crohn's disease or the sexually acquired reactive arthritis group. The presence of sore eyes may aid in the diagnosis: this may be due to uveitis or conjunctivitis as seen in Reiter's syndrome or Behçet's syndrome. Both diseases are associated with the involvement of a single joint, but occasionally by symmetrical arthritis. A history of attacks in one big toe followed by symmetrical arthritis may raise the possibility of gout or pseudogout as an underlying cause. Back pain has to be taken into account particularly if one is trying to exclude sero-negative arthritis. The presence of diarrhoea is also worth eliciting by direct questioning in order to exclude the arthritic reactions, particularly to such organisms as *Salmonella, Shigella* or *Yersinia*. Infective arthritis may be symmetrical although it is more commonly monoarticular. A history of skin rash may be helpful in the diagnosis of psoriatic arthritis and this should certainly be considered if there is a history of nail changes with pitting or ridging even in the absence of skin lesions. Occupational history or sporting history can sometimes yield useful information, for example 'wicket keeper's hands' can give symmetrical arthritis of the small joints in the hand, and 'fast bowler's ankles' certainly lead to bilateral arthritis of the ankles, both of these giving rise to osteoarthritis. Osteoarthritis may cause symmetrical polyarthritis of the knees.

EXAMINATION

A full medical examination should be carried out. First of all, the swollen joints should be looked at and then examined for presence of effusion. A further search should be made of all the joints, including those of the spine, to exclude other coincidental joint pathology of which the patient may or may not have complained. The skin should be examined for evidence of psoriatic plaques; classically these may occur on extensor surfaces of the elbows and knees, but they may also occur in the most unlikely places such as the scalp or pubic hair and may be absent altogether, the only vestiges of psoriasis being the presence of pits and ridging on nails. Examination of the spine should include the cervical spine as this may be the only evidence of arthritis of the spine, particularly in women with ankylosing spondylitis or both women and men with psoriatic spondylitis. It is worth looking at the eyes for uveitis, or even looking for the dry eyes or dry mouth of Sjögren's syndrome which is associated with many of the causes of polyarthritis, particularly rheumatoid arthritis, systemic lupus erythematosus

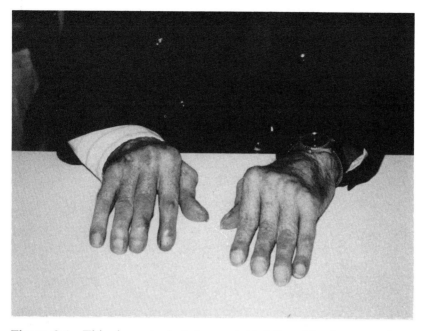

Figure 3.1 This shows typical rheumatoid deformities (swan neck deformities of the fingers and Z deformities of the thumbs) in a patient with nodular erosive rheumatoid arthritis.

(SLE) and polyarthritis nodosa. A search of the skin is also necessary to exclude rheumatoid nodules which may occur anywhere rather than just the classical sites of elbows and knees: the author has seen them on the buttocks and in the hair. Sometimes minute nodules may be found on the elbows of patients with SLE. Tophi should also be looked for in the pinnae of the ears or on the nails or pulps of the fingers, these are indicative of the presence of chronic tophaceous gout. Balanitis should be sought by examination of the genitalia as should ulceration. The mouth should be looked at for evidence of buccal ulceration as with Behçet's syndrome or Henoch–Schönlein purpura. A rash across the face may be present in patients with SLE. Erythema marginatum should be sought over the thighs and buttocks to exclude the diagnosis of rheumatic fever; a search should also be made of the nail beds for evidence of

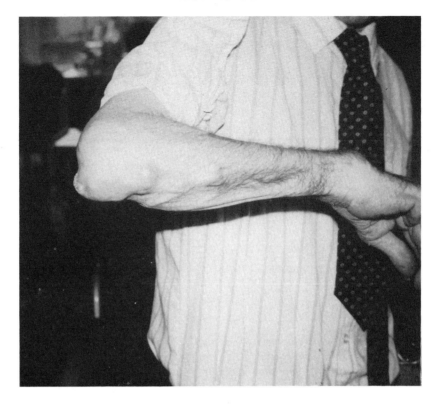

Figure 3.2   Rheumatoid nodules on the elbows and forearm.

vascular lesions which may be found either in association with bacterial endocarditis or rheumatoid arthritis or even SLE.

INVESTIGATIONS

Investigations may well give the answer very easily. The presence of an elevated serum acid level may aid diagnosis, but is not in itself diagnostic of gout and the only way to be certain of the diagnosis is by aspiration and the use of a polarized microscope (see Chapter 11 on gout). Pseudogout is clearly diagnosed by the same man-

18

oeuvre. Infection should be excluded by aspiration and a search under the microscope for organisms using a Gram or Ziehl–Neelsen stain, and culture may be indicated as well. A rheumatoid factor test is found to be positive in 70–80% of patients with rheumatoid arthritis. An antinuclear test is invariably but not always positive in SLE, but the DNA binding is nearly always positive. Sometimes patients with SLE may have antibodies such as anti-Ro or anti-La: Jo-1 is found in patients with dermatomyositis. Mixed connective tissue disease may be something of a diagnostic dilemma, having some but not all features of many of the diseases already outlined. Here extractable nuclear antigens may be found on immunological testing. Blood cultures may give further information with regard to the possibility of infection, and an ASO titre is helpful to exclude bacterial endocarditis or rheumatic fever. The diagnosis of polyarteritis nodosa, another cause of symmetrical arthritis, is extremely difficult to make. It tends to be more a diagnosis of exclusion by investigation, the only definitive way being to look for aneurysmal dilatation of the renal arteries by means of a renal arteriogram and this in itself is rarely indicated clinically.

MANAGEMENT

The treatment of osteoarthritis involves the use of analgesics and non-steroidal anti-inflammatory drugs (see Chapter 13). Bilateral osteoarthritis of the knees in a sportsman may be an indication to persuade the patient to give up that aspect of the sport. A simple explanation that going on with it will simply lead eventually to a loss of joint space and more severe problems may be enough to alert the patient to the problems that he himself is creating: it is good being a fast bowler at 45, but there is an argument for switching to spin bowling if it means not wearing the joints out! In most cases of osteoarthritis of the hip or knee, a walking stick used in the opposite hand is far superior to any drug. Surgery may be needed in advanced cases.

The management of rheumatoid arthritis involves treating the acute disease with bed rest, splinting, passive movements by physiotherapists and non-steroidal anti-inflammatory drugs to overcome the acute phase. The management of chronic rheumatoid disease involves non-steroidal anti-inflammatory drugs, and in some patients disease modifying antirheumatic therapy. The decision about this is in all probability one that should be made by the hospital consultant in conjunction with the general practitioner rather than by the general practitioner alone, and monitoring is very much a combined operation. The disease modifying antirheumatic drugs, whilst they are useful for the condition and bring about long periods of remission from symptoms in some patients, are less successful for others. For these patients it may be necessary to embark on the use of immunosuppressive drugs. Intravenous methyl-prednisolone infusions plus cyclophosphamide may be indicated for the severe cases of crumbling, often found in late middle-age, late onset rheumatoid arthritis which are associated with a bad prognosis in terms of the articular manifestations. Treatment of the extra-articular manifestations of rheumatoid arthritis involves the use of immunosuppressive therapy and sometimes corticosteroids. Life-threatening conditions in particular, for example pulmonary fibrosis, may be treated by this combination.

The articular manifestations of SLE are best treated by non-steroidal anti-inflammatory drugs. The use of immunosuppressive plus or minus steroids for neurological or renal lesions is beyond the scope of this chapter.

The treatment of gout is discussed in Chapter 11, but is basically the treatment of the acute attack with non-steroidal anti-inflammatory drugs such as indomethacin, piroxicam or naproxen. The indication for the use of a long-acting antigout agent such as allopurinol is the occurrence of two or more attacks over a short space of time, where a long-acting drug can be said to be less of a burden if taken regularly than the disease itself. The disease may lead to the presence of renal calculi and for this reason antigout therapy should be given early rather than late. If the patient is overweight, dieting to reduce weight may be as helpful as the use of an antigout agent.

The treatment of acute painful joints as seen in rheumatic fever or bacterial endocarditis is bed rest, splinting and the use of soluble aspirin, and in the presence of infection an appropriate oral antibiotic.

CARCINOMA POLYARTHRITIS

A polyarthritis resembling rheumatoid arthritis is occasionally the presenting manifestation of malignancy. The diagnosis of carcinoma polyarthritis requires a temporal relationship between the onset of the arthritis and the discovery of tumour; hypertrophic, osteoarthropathy and metastatic involvement of the synovium or periarticular bone must be excluded. Its differentiation from rheumatoid arthritis is summarized in Table 3.1.

Table 3.1 *Differentiation between rheumatoid arthritis and carcinoma polyarthritis*

	RA	CP
Age at onset	Middle age	Elderly
Joint involvement	Symmetrical	Asymmetrical
Pattern of joint involvement	Small joints and other joints in upper and lower limb	Joints of lower extremity, spares the small joint
RF	Positive (80%)	Negative
Rheumatoid nodules	Present	Abent
Family history	Positive	Negative

Table 3.2 *Diagnostic criteria for rheumatoid arthritis (ARA)*

A. **Classical Rheumatoid Arthritis**

This diagnosis requires seven of the following criteria:

1 to 5: the joint signs or symptoms must be continuous for at least six weeks. Any one of the features listed under exclusions will exclude a patient from this and all other categories.

Criteria 2, 3, 4, 5 and 6 should have been observed by a physician.

1. Morning stiffness
2. Pain or motion or tenderness in at least one joint
3. Swelling (soft tissue or fluid not bony) in at least one joint
4. Swelling of at least one other joint
5. Symmetric joint swelling with simultaneous involvement of the same joint on both sides of the body (terminal interphalangeal joint involvement will not satisfy this criteria)
6. Subcutaneous nodules
7. X-ray changes typical of rheumatoid arthritis which must include at least periarticular osteoporosis
8. Positive rheumatoid factor by any method
9. Poor mucin precipitate from synovial fluid
10. Characteristic histological changes in synovium
11. Characteristic histological changes in nodules

B. **Definite Rheumatoid Arthritis**

This diagnosis requires five of the above criteria:
In criteria 1 to 5 the joint signs or symptoms must be continuous for at least six weeks.

C. **Probable Rheumatoid Arthritis**

This diagnosis requires three of the above criteria:
In criteria 1 to 5 the joint signs or symptoms must be continuous for at least six weeks.

D. **Possible Rheumatoid Arthritis**

This diagnosis requires two of the following criteria and total duration of joint symptoms must be at least three months:

1. Morning stiffness
2. Tenderness or pain on motion (observed by physician) with history of recurrence or persistence for three weeks
3. History or observation of joint swelling
4. Subcutaneous nodules
4. High ESR or C reactive protein

E. **Exclusions**

1. Typical rash of SLE (Malar erythema or discoid LE)
2. High concentration of LE cells
3. Histological evidence of polyarteritis nodosa
4. Dermatomyositis
5. ? Scleroderma
6. Rheumatic fever
7. Gouty arthritis
8. Tophi
9. Clinical picture characteristic of acute infective arthritis of bacterial or viral origin
10. Tuberculous arthritis
11. Reiter's syndrome
12. Shoulder hand syndrome
13. Hypertrophic osteoarthropathy
14. Neuropathic joints
15. Homogentisic aciduria
16. Sarcoidosis
17. Multiple myeloma
18. Erythema nodosum
19. Leukemia or lymphoma
20. Agammaglobulinaemia

4

Early Morning Stiffness

□ □ □ □ □ □ □ □ □ □ □ □ □

It is necessary to establish what is meant by early morning stiffness. There are two types: the first is mild and does not prevent the patient getting up and performing his daily activities. It is really inactivity stiffness and is frequently found in patients with osteoarthritis, usually involving the hands and possibly the feet. The second type is severe and frustrating: the patient cannot move or get out of bed and is unable to perform his daily activities, life is very much affected by the stiffness until it wears off. This is the problem that is encountered in polymyositis, polymyalgia rheumatica and certain rheumatic diseases.

Table 4.1 *Differential diagnosis of early morning stiffness*

Rheumatoid arthritis
Osteoarthritis
Polymyositis
Polymyalgia rheumatica
Psoriatic arthropathy
Underlying neoplasia
Mixed connective tissue disease

HISTORY

Mild early morning stiffness is in reality a feature of ageing. Most patients who develop osteoarthritis have mild underlying early morning stiffness, and give a history of stiffness rather than pain first thing in the morning when they awake and sometimes in the night, but rapidly wearing off when they sit up; they are then able to get up and perform their normal everyday tasks. Patients sometimes find it difficult to distinguish between stiffness and pain, often lumping the two things together.

The more profound type of early morning stiffness is a major problem as it can last certainly up to midday, and the patient may well be confined to bed for this time. Sitting up may be impossible. Clearly a history should involve any history of polyarthritis and any indication of the seronegative markers (see Chapter 5 on seronegative arthritis). In patients over the age of 50, polymyalgia rheumatica and temporal arteritis are not uncommon. Polymyalgia rheumatica presents with extreme incapacitating morning stiffness, the patients having this as their only symptom, with no history of joint involvement. Temporal arteritis may present in the same way and the diagnosis can only be made on the basis of investigation. Other patients with temporal arteritis will present with unilateral headache and complain of pain over the temporal artery area. These patients can occasionally complain of claudication as well. Patients with severe muscle pain which is disabling and who exhibit weakness may have polymyositis. Neurological diseases can sometimes present with severe intractable stiffness which is not really true stiffness but is a feature of generalized weakness. Cervical myelopathy can also present in this way, giving stiffness particularly in the upper arms and pain down the arms. If the symptoms are unilateral it may make the diagnosis easier, particularly if the patient complains of unilateral weakness.

EXAMINATION

The finding of weakness and tenderness clearly indicates pathology. The presence of tenderness over the temporal arteries may well lead to the diagnosis of temporal arteritis. Neurological signs should be sought, particularly plantar responses that have become extensor, or upper motor neurone lesions suggestive of cervical myelopathy. The joints should be checked for any evidence of either rheumatoid arthritis, seronegative markers or osteoarthritis. Wasting should be sought in particular with reference to Pancoast tumours of the lungs, where a frequent finding is of wasting of the intrinsic muscles of the hand, often unilaterally, along with Horner's syndrome.

INVESTIGATIONS

An ESR may be extremely helpful. A normal ESR may well exclude or make very unlikely such diseases as polymyalgia rheumatica and temporal arteritis. It would also make diagnoses such as rheumatoid arthritis and seronegative arthritis less likely. It will not exclude underlying nuerological disease or cervical myelopathy. In order to exclude the diagnosis of temporal arteritis, a temporal artery biopsy may be indicated. It has to be of a reasonable size and the histology has to be sought extensively in order to exclude the skip lesions which are found on the pathological sectioning. Cervical myelopathy may be partly excluded by flexion and extension and AP and lateral views of the cervical spine. This may not be enough, myelography being indicated in order to show a true block. In order to exclude such conditions as polymyositis, it is necessary to undertake an electromyogram (EMG), the purpose of which is to demonstrate large polyphasic activity in the muscles which is compatible with this condition. Serum creatine phosphokinase (CPK) is very high. In order to confirm this diagnosis it may be necessary to carry out a muscle biopsy.

MANAGEMENT

Management of this condition again involves taking a full history, carrying out a full examination and making an accurate diagnosis. If the diagnosis is simply osteoarthritis, then the use of a non-steroidal anti-inflammatory drug may be extremely efficient in relieving the mild early morning stiffness along with the painful joints. If the condition is rheumatoid arthritis, then indomethacin particularly given as either a suppository last thing at night, or 100 mg orally nocte is also excellent at relieving symptoms.

Polymyalgia rheumatica and temporal arteritis once diagnosed should be treated aggressively, the former with at least 20 mg of prednisolone and the latter with 40 mg of prednisolone, the aim being to rapidly reduce the dosage to around 10 mg daily and then more slowly. The object is to reduce the dose by $2\frac{1}{2}$ mg every two weeks down to 10 mg, and then monthly from there on. This is a difficult condition to treat; there have been relapses on withdrawal of the drug in patients who are asymptomatic with a normal ESR. These are, however, rare and the outlined policy will treat most patients with this condition. With some patients it may well be up to 8 years before it is possible to wean the patients off the steroids completely. To withhold steroids in this condition may be extremely hazardous as in the presence of the polymyalgia syndrome some patients do indeed develop temporal arteritis and there is a risk that these patients can go blind unless the steroid is employed.

The sero-negative arthritides are discussed in Chapter 5: specifically a non-steroidal anti-inflammatory drug such as indomethacin is highly effective at reducing early morning stiffness in these patients.

Whether or not patients with polymyositis should be subjected to a search for primary tumour is a controversial area. Depending on which series is read, the incidence of tumour varies between 10% and 50%, but is somewhat similar to looking for a needle in a haystack. It is in all probability worth carrying out a barium meal and an IVP. There are those who also feel that a CT scan to check for lymph node enlargement of the posterior abdominal wall or pancreatic neoplasms is worth carrying out. Whether these investigations are all entirely cost-effective and in the patient's interest is another matter. Excision of a primary tumour may lead to regression of the profound stiffness, but this is not always the case and the results from this procedure are sometimes extremely disappointing. It used to be said that the use of steroids in polymyositis in the presence of tumour did not relieve the symptoms, but in the absence of tumour did: this is again a myth which has proved not to be true in practice. However, polymyositis is best treated with corticosteroids as this seems to reduce the inflammatory component of the muscle symptoms and allows the patient to resume some activity. Physiotherapy is clearly of importance here to try and make the best use of what muscle power is available to the patient.

RARE CAUSES

Several syndromes consisting of progessive muscular rigidity have been described and can be grossly classified into:

(1)   Myogenic syndromes:
        e.g. myotonia congenita
              myotonia dystrophica.

(2)   Neuromyogenic syndromes:
        e.g. stiffman syndrome
              Isaac's syndrome.

Neuromyogenic syndromes usually present with generalized muscle stiffness.

Table 4.2   Diagnosis and treatment of neuromyogenic syndromes

	Isaac's syndrome	*Stiffman syndrome*
Sleep or general anaesthesia	Persistent stiffness	Stiffness abolished
Diazepam	Persistent stiffness	Stiffness abolished
Phenytoin	Stiffness abolished	Persistent stiffness

5

The Seronegative Spondarthropathies

□ □ □ □ □ □ □ □ □ □ □ □ □

A patient with one of the seronegative arthritic conditions may present with back pain accompanied by other features which suggest an alternative diagnosis to that of simple back strain. A careful history and examination may be very revealing

HISTORY

First of all the back. Is there morning stiffness? Is the pain confined to the lumber spine? Is there also neck involvement? The sex of the patient is relevant; these conditions, particularly ankylosing spondylitis, are more common in the male than the female. However, when occurring in young females the symptoms are often present in the neck rather than the lower lumbar spine, and a persistent history of neck pain in a young woman should be treated as suspicious of underlying ankylosing spondylitis. It is unusual for ankylosing spondylitis to be associated with sciatica, the presence of which should suggest another diagnosis. Often the stiffness passes off during the day, and exercise may well relieve it.

Other systemic enquiries

A variety of conditions other than ankylosing spondylitis can be associated with sacro-iliitis. Uveitis is a common feature of this group of conditions and may point in this direction: it may occur before, at the same time or after the problems with the back. A careful history of skin lesions on elbows or knees may indicate psoriasis, and a family history of psoriasis may be helpful. In the absence of skin changes, nail changes alone may be enough to make the diagnosis, and the patient may complain of ridging or pitting of the nails in the absence of other features.

Diarrhoea may be a presenting feature. This problem is found in 10% of patients with ankylosing spondylitis; on the other hand Crohn's disease, ulcerative colitis and infective gut disease due to *Salmonella, Shigella, Yersinia, Campylobacter* or other organisms can present in this way. A history of painful buccal or genital ulceration with arthritis may point to the diagnosis of Behçet's syndrome. Similar buccal ulcerations occur in Reiter's syndrome but are painless. A history of urethral discharge along with uveitis and arthritis should suggest Reiter's syndrome. Sometimes this can exist in incomplete forms: an example would be urethritis along with the sacro-iliitis. This so-called 'incomplete' Reiter's syndrome is better called sexually-acquired reactive arthropathy or SARA.

Table 5.1 *The spondarthropathies*

---

1. Ankylosing spondylitis
2. Reiter's syndrome
3. Sexually acquired reactive arthropathy
4. Psoriatic arthropathy
5. Arthritis associated with chronic inflammatory bowel disease
6. Reactive arthritis associated with infective gut disease
7. ? Behçet's syndrome

EXAMINATION

A full and careful examination should involve the back to check for movement, stiffness of the lumbar spine and immobility in flexion and extension being common features. Lateral movements are often very restricted. The cervical spine and the thoracic spine may also be involved in this condition and limitation of movement may be panspinous.

The eyes should be checked for presence of uveitis (they would appear sore and red with ciliary injection). The body, skin and hair should be checked for presence of psoriatic plaques. A single plaque occurring in the scalp may be enough to make the diagnosis in the absence of the classic findings of psoriasis on the extensor surfaces of the elbows and knees. Pitting and ridging of the nails in the absence of skin disease may also indicate psoriasis.

Examination of the joints may reveal a variety of different sorts of arthropathy. This can vary from single or asymmetrical peripheral joint involvement to a symmetrical rheumatoid-like pattern, or there may be symmetrical terminal joint involvement. Occasionally the arthritis may be confined to single large joints, in particular the knee with Reiter's syndrome. One may see arthritis of the big toe 'metatarso-phalangeal joint' as in gout and small joints of the feet which is classically found in association with sexually acquired reactive arthritis, or with ulcerative colitis or Crohn's disease.

The presence of peripheral joint arthritis is an aid to diagnosis particularly in terms of its pattern of distribution. Occasionally, the arthritis of psoriasis may become extremely severe leading to mutilans deformity with 'concertinaring' of the hands and gross destruction of the joints with eventual total loss of function. This is fortunately a rare complication.

Examination of the gut using sigmoidscopy may reveal proctitis of the granular type or may even reveal the presence of bloody mucosa, suggesting ulcerative colitic lesions. Urethral examination in a male is easy and may reveal the presence of either ulcers or a urethral discharge. It may be necessary to evoke the help of the venerologist to exclude urethral problems completely. The diagnosis of urethritis on clinical examination in a woman is extremely difficult, and it is more common to see cervicitis rather than a true urethritis.

Table 5.2 *Types of psoriatic arthritis*

1. Arthritis of the distal interphalangeal joints
2. Asymmetric pauci-articular (less than 4) arthritis
3. Symmetric seronegative polyarthritis
4. Arthritis mutilans
5. Sacro-iliitis and bamboo spine

INVESTIGATIONS

X-rays of the sacro-iliac joints are helpful, but there are pitfalls for the unwary. Young patients often have blurring of the sacro-iliac joints as do women, and in both these groups it is often difficult to interpret abnormality in X-rays. Sclerosis is an early sign of impending change: blurring and erosions are seen and eventually fusion occurs. Sacro-ilitis itself does not lead to the diagnosis of ankylosing spondylitis but is a feature of a group of diseases including ankylosing spondylitis. An X-ray of the lumbar spine will reveal squaring of the vertebrae, syndesmophyte formation and bony ridging. Bony ridging can be panspinous leading to the so-called bamboo spine. Occasionally an erosion may be seen on the anterior surface of a vertebra, the so-called Romanus lesion, which is in fact an erosive change. X-rays of the peripheral joints when they are involved may reveal erosions but these are relatively mild compared with the arthritis which is present, as distinct from rheumatoid arthritis where the erosions and the severity often go hand in hand. In psoriatic arthropathy a 'pencil and egg-cup' deformity is sometimes encountered, this is tapering of a metatarsal bone followed by widening and splaying of a proximal interphalangeal bone at the metacarpalphalangeal joint.

Laboratory investigations include the ESR which is often an unhelpful guide here. One can encounter highly active ankylosing spondylitis with a normal ESR or mild disease associated with a very high ESR. Anaemia is often encountered in all these diseases, as is a raised white cell count in conditions associated with an infective component.

Stools should be examined for blood and bacteria, although it may be necessary to carry out specific antibody tests to exclude *Salmonella, Shigella Yersinia* and *Campylobacter* infections.

Whilst primarily still a research tool, tissue typing is of value. Where there is doubt about the appearance of sacro-iliac joints, a tissue typing that shows HLA-B27 supports the diagnosis of ankylosing spondylitis. Cases of ankylosing spondylitis occur with a negative HLA-B27 tissue type but this is unusual, 96% of all patients being HLA-B27 positive. 50% of patients who have Reiter's syndrome are HLA-B27 positive.

Further investigations

A barium meal with follow-through examination and a barium enema may be necessary to exclude Crohn's disease or ulcerative colitis, and a rectal biopsy may give tissue diagnosis. There is no definite test for Reiter's syndrome, diagnosis of which is made on the basis of history and examination. The finding of elevated and changing titres of *Chlamydia* antibodies is a research tool and is not applicable to clinical disease monitoring. There is no diagnostic test for Behçet's syndrome. However, 50% of patients with this syndrome exhibit a cutaneous phenomenon termed 'pathergy'; venipuncture or injection of sterile saline into the skin results in a pustule formation. The diagnosis is based on clinical examination which has to exclude other causes of ulcers such as *Herpes simplex* virus.

MANAGEMENT

The emphasis in the management of ankylosing spondylitis and other causes of sacro-iliitis with involvement of the spine is on physiotherapy. This should be taught to the patient, carried out by the patient himself and rigorously supported by doctor, nurse and physiotherapist alike. The aim is to keep the patient as mobile as possible for as long as possible. Corsets, plaster jackets and other means of stopping movement are to be avoided. A careful explanation of exercising through the pain and of using non-steroidal anti-inflammatory drugs to relieve pain in an 'on demand' way should be given to the patient. This approach with positive support is the best way to keep the patient mobile. In the event of the patient becoming less mobile, there is an argument for using a swimming pool, local pools being as good as hospital departments. This is particularly applicable when there is panspinous involvement.

The treatment of psoriatic arthropathy along with spondylitis is by means of non-steroidal anti-inflammatory drugs for the majority of cases. For some, disease-modifying drugs such as azathioprine, methotrexate or chlorambucil (in very severe exceptional cases) may be indicated.

Treatment of Reiter's syndrome is by the use of an appropriate tetracycline-like antibiotic to eradicate any infecting agents such as *Chlamydia*. Treatment of underlying ulcerative colitis or Crohn's disease depends on the severity of the condition: the use of azathioprine now appears to have much support with the occasional use of corticosteroid enemas. Treatment of underlying bowel infection is by the use of an appropriate antibiotic.

The prognosis for ankylosing spondylitis with enthusiastic support is good, but the patient himself is his own boss and only if the condition is clearly explained, the right treatment given and the right attitudes conveyed, can the patient then make a suitable therapeutic response.

6

Paediatric Rheumatism

□ □ □ □ □ □ □ □ □ □ □ □

Musculoskeletal complaints are common in children. Worried parents often consult their general practitioner because of the shape of their child's feet and legs and the way he or she walks. The feet of newborn babies look flat and continue to do so when they start to stand up by the end of the first year. By the third year, the feet begin to develop a normal plantar arch.

Babies and toddlers have bow legs; when the feet are together, the knees may be up to 5 cm apart. The knees become knocked by the third to fourth years of life; the intermalleolar distance may be up to 5 cm when the child stands up with his knees together, and may be even greater in obese children. The legs should, however, be straight by the age of 11 to 12 years. If the bowing or the knocking of the knees is asymmetrical or greater than normal, a specialist opinion should be sought. An extreme degree of bowing in an Asian baby raises the suspicion of rickets.

CAUSES

Trauma

Musculoskeletal trauma in children may manifest itself in fractures, ligamentous strain or even cartilage injury.

Table 6.1 *Causes of painful limp*

1. Trauma
2. Perthes' disease
3. Slipped upper femoral epiphysis
4. Osteoid osteoma
5. Transient synovitis of the hip
6. Septic arthritis
7. Osteochondroses
8. Other inflammatory arthritides (CJA)
9. Minor conditions e.g. warts

Table 6.2 *Causes of painless limp*

1. Leg inequality
2. Neuro-muscular disorders e.g. cerebral palsy and muscular dystrophy
3. Hysteria

Juvenile osteochondroses and chondromalacia patellae

Idiopathic osteonecrosis of the proximal femoral epiphysis (Perthes' disease) may be suspected in boys aged 3–12 years with hip pain and a limp.

Knee pain in children aged 10–15 years could be due to defective ossification of the tibial tuberosity (Osgood–Schlatter's disease) or the lower half of the patella (Sinding–Larsen disease), or to softening and erosion of the articular cartilage of the patella (chondromalacia patellae), especially in girls and cyclists. These three conditions are benign and the parents and child should be reassured. Rest is imposed if pain is severe and analgesics are prescribed. These conditions tend to resolve spontaneously within 6–18 months.

Infections

Various upper respiratory tract infections can give rise to arthralgia, but arthritis can develop during an infection with rubella, mumps, chickenpox, adenovirus, hepatitis B and *Mycoplasma*. Gonococcal arthritis should be suspected in teenagers. Septic arthritis should always be thought of in systemically ill children with hot painful swollen joints.

Acute osteomyelitis is more common in boys than girls and should be suspected in a child with a high temperature and localized pain. Localized bone tenderness strongly supports the diagnosis. Tuberculosis of bone and joints, though less common, can cause severe deformities and disability if not diagnosed and treated early.

Malignancy

Leukaemia, neuroblastoma, Hodgkin's and non-Hodgkin's lymphoma and other forms of malignant tumour can cause and present with musculoskeletal pain mimicking arthritis; these should always be suspected when the pain is severe and the child looks systemically ill.

Collagen/vascular disease

Systemic lupus erythematosus, dermatomyositis, polyarteritis nodosa, Wegener's granuloma, mucocutaneous lymph node syndrome (Kawasaki syndrome) and Henoch–Schönlein purpura can present with arthralgia, polyarthritis or even a single hot swollen joint accompanying a skin rash.

Blood disease

Haemophilia, Christmas disease, sickle-cell disease, thrombocytopenia purpura (idiopathic or secondary) and other blood diseases may present with a single or multiple hot swollen joints. Aspiration is helpful in establishing a diagnosis.

Reiter's syndrome and reactive arthritis

Classical Reiter's syndrome (a triad of urethritis or colitis, conjunctivitis and arthritis) is rare in children, but 'incomplete' reactive arthritis (sometimes called incomplete Reiter's syndrome, or more commonly reactive arthritis) occurs in teenagers following infection with *Shigella, Yersinia, Campylobacter, Salmonella, Neisseria gonorrhoeae* and chronic meningococcaemia. The arthritis is sterile and mainly affects large joints such as knees, hips, ankles, elbows and wrists. About 50% of patients carry the HLA-B27 antigen.

The condition has a good prognosis responding favourably to rest and non-steroidal anti-inflammatory drugs, the majority of cases resolving within 3–9 months. Only rarely are deformities seen. Very occasionally the condition recurs or there may even be multiple relapses or remissions.

Rheumatic fever

Rheumatic fever is one of the poststreptococcal diseases and is a rarity in the Western World nowadays, being found more commonly in the Third World. Its five major manifestations include carditis (endocarditis, myocarditis and/or pericarditis), polyarthritis, chorea, erythema marginatum (evanescent erythematous non-pruritic rash mainly on the trunk) and subcutaneous nodules. The arthritis is the commonest feature and mainly affects the joints of the lower limbs: the onset is abrupt and signs of inflammation are florid within 24 hours. The affected joint subsides and at the same time one or two others become inflamed, hence the term migratory arthritis. Permanent deformities are rare. The minor manifestations include fever, arthralgia and previous history of rheumatic fever or rheumatic heart disease.

The diagnosis of rheumatic fever is highly probable if in addition to evidence of preceding streptococcal infection (increased anti-streptolysin 'O' titre or other streptococcal antibodies, positive throat culture for Lancefield group A β-haemolytic streptococcus, or recent scarlet fever), two major features or one major and two minor features are present.

Treatment is symptomatic with rest and salicylates. A 10-day course of penicillin should be given and a monthly intramuscular injection of 1.2 million units of benzathine penicillin G should be continued for life.

Table 6.3 *Jones criteria (revised) for guidance in the diagnosis of rheumatic fever*

Major	*Minor*
Carditis	Clinical fever
Polyarthritis	Arthralgia
Chorea	Previous rheumatic fever or
Erythema marginatum	rheumatic heart disease
Subcutaneous nodules	

Plus

Supporting evidence of preceeding streptococcal infection: increased ASO, positive throat culture for group A streptococcus or recent scarlet fever

2 major or 1 major and 2 minor criteria indicate a high probability of rheumatic fever if supported by evidence of a preceding streptococcal infection.

CHRONIC JUVENILE ARTHRITIS

Having excluded the previously mentioned diseases in a patient with persistent arthritis of at least six weeks' duration in one or more joints, the child is said to suffer from chronic juvenile arthritis which includes Still's disease (three types), sero-positive juvenile rheumatoid arthritis, juvenile ankylosing spondylitis, psoriatic arthritis and arthritis associated with inflammatory bowel disease (see Table 6.4). The latter four diseases tend to occur later in childhood, while Still's disease tends to affect children below the age of five (except the polyarticular type which can occur at any age). Amyloidosis may be a later complication.

Still's disease

There are three main types of Still's disease: systemic, polyarticular and pauciarticular.

The systemic type characteristically presents with high intermittent fever accompanied by an evanescent non-pruritic urticaria-like rash occurring mainly on the trunk and proximal parts of the limbs. Other features include pleurisy, pericarditis, hepatosplenomegaly (which may be extreme) and lymphadenopathy. The joint manifestations may be minimal and may appear much later in the disease course. The child becomes anaemic and has a neutrophil leukocytosis. The rheumatoid factor and antinuclear antibodies are negative. Half the affected children suffer relapses.

In the polyarticular type which mainly affects girls, the above manifestations are much less evident but the joint manifestations are florid. The joints are usually symmetrically affected, including the small joints of the hands and feet as well as the larger joints. Hip disease is common (40%) and usually disabling. The neck is frequently affected and may fuse easily in the disease. The temporo-mandibular joint may be involved leading to lower jaw recession. Radiologically, subperiosteal bone formation may be seen in relationship to inflamed joints but erosions are late to develop. The rheumatoid factor is negative but antinuclear antibodies may be positive in 25% of patients. Bone growth is usually stunted resulting in short stature with short fingers and toes, fused short neck and receding chin. However, the overall prognosis is better than that for juvenile sero-positive rheumatoid arthritis.

In the pauciarticular type, again mainly affecting girls, large joints are affected (usually knees, ankles and elbows) and the hips are mostly spared. By definition, four or less joints are affected during the first six months of the disease. More important, half the patients develop iridocyclitis which is often insidious and chronic, and may be complicated by the secondary development of posterior synechiae, cataract, glaucoma and band keratopathy; hence blindness. These children are sero-negative for rheumatoid factor and half are positive for the antinuclear antibodies.

Juvenile rheumatoid arthritis

This occurs in older children, mainly girls, and its course and treatment resembles the adult type. All the children are sero-positive for rheumatoid factor and 75% have positive antinuclear antibodies. Half the children end up with destroyed joints.

Juvenile ankylosing spondylitis

This condition affects older boys and its course and management is similar to the adult type. 10% of these children develop a painful red eye (acute iridocyclitis). 75% of the children are HLA-B27 positive, and antinuclear antibodies and rheumatoid factor are both negative.

Management of chronic juvenile arthritis

The aim of management of children with chronic juvenile arthritis is to allow the child to lead as normal a life as possible with minimal disability. This is best achieved in a specialist unit and requires in addition to the multi-professional team (occupational therapist, physiotherapist, psychologist, orthotist, etc.), the co-operation of the child's parent or teacher. The involvement of the general practitioner is vital; he can look after the child between hospital visits as well as help to organize the services required.

Treatment begins with education of the parents and gaining their confidence as their co-operation can affect the outcome of rehabilitation favourably. The school teacher also needs to be informed and educated about this disease. The Arthritis and Rheumatism Council booklets on chronic juvenile arthritis are very helpful.

During the acute phase of the disease, the child has to be admitted to hospital and kept in bed with splinting of the hands, knees and feet to prevent deformity. The child also needs to lie prone for 10–15 minutes four times a day to prevent hip deformities. Aspirin is still the drug of choice in doses of 80 mg kg^{-1} d^{-1} in divided doses: if there is inadequate response the dose may be raised to 120 mg kg^{-1} d^{-1}. Serum salicylate levels should be repeated regularly and the dose kept in the therapeutic range of 20–30 mg/100 ml. If aspirin cannot be tolerated, naproxen or ibuprofen may be used.

Once the acute phase has subsided, the physiotherapist can teach the patient various exercises to strengthen his muscles and improve the range of movement in his joints. The hydrotherapy pool is useful in this respect. The occupational therapist can help the child to overcome any difficulties with daily activities with the use of training, aids and modification of the home.

If the disease is severe and continues to be active, then gold, penicillamine or hydroxychloroquine may be used. Corticosteroids are used if there is no response to these drugs; however, steroids are indicated when there is iridocyclitis. Side effects of steroids are many: stunting of growth, muscle wasting, osteoporosis, glucose intolerance, trunk obesity, etc. Alternateday steroids may produce fewer side effects, particularly on growth.

Four-monthly visits to the ophthalmologist are vital for early detection and treatment of iridocyclitis.

Six-monthly reviews of the patient in a combined clinic with a rheumatologist and an orthopaedic surgeon should be undertaken to consider any surgical procedure (e.g. synovectomy, soft tissue release, etc.) which may help to improve the patient's functional disability or even his appearance.

When the child leaves school he may need vocational advice.

Table 6.4 *Chronic juvenile arthritis*

	Age at onset	Sex ratio	Laboratory tests	Other features
Still's disease Systemic type	under 5	almost equal	ANA neg RF neg	Fever, rash, polyserositis, hepatosplenomegaly: lymphadenopathy, anaemia, leukocytosis
Still's disease Polyarticular	any age	90% girls	ANA pos 25% RF neg	Any joint affected including neck. Destructive arthritis in 15%. Hip disease common
Still's disease Mono- or pauciarticular	under 5	90% girls	ANA pos 50% RF neg	Chronic iridocyclitis 50%. Affects knees, ankles, elbows but not usually hips
Juvenile rheumatoid arthritis	late childhood	80% girls	ANA pos 75% RF pos 100%	Resembles adult RA. Destructive arthritis in 50%
Juvenile ankylosing spondylitis	late childhood	90% boys	ANA neg RF neg HLA-B27 pos 75%	Resembles adult AS. Acute iridocyclitis
Psoriatic arthritis	late childhood	F>M	ANA neg RF neg	Psoriasis may follow the arthritis after years. DIP usually involved.
Colitic arthritis	late childhood	equal	ANA neg RF neg	Two types: 1) spondylitic 2) large peripheral joints

7

Back Pain

☐ ☐ ☐ ☐ ☐ ☐ ☐ ☐ ☐ ☐ ☐ ☐ ☐

Back pain is the commonest problem of a rheumatological nature to confront the general practitioner. It is said that some 64 million days of work are lost per annum in the United Kingdom as a result of this predicament: it is therefore second only to bronchitis as a cause of lost working time. There are 1.5 million new patient GP consultations a year, and 5 million total GP consultations. The majority of patients with back pain will recover from their problems. One survey suggests that 98% will have lost their symptoms within 3 months of onset; this is based on a hospital survey and therefore was a selected population of patients bad enough to present to hospital outpatient departments. The aim of this chapter therefore is to try and give some guidelines as to which patients should be referred to hospital and what points should be sought in history and examination to suggest underlying problems beyond the simple mechanical type.

One way of thinking of back pain is to consider age related to causes. It is unusual for children to have backache; minor degrees of spina bifida probably do not cause this problem at this stage, presenting symptomatically only later in life. Sportsmen and the young active adult can develop spondylolysis and spondylolisthesis. The more mature adult may develop ankylosing spondylitis and the associated sacroilitis plus other types of sero-negative arthropathy, in particular Reiter's syndrome. It is worth remembering that there is a group of seemingly unrelated conditions which can produce sacroilitis (see Chapter 5 on sero-negative arthritis). Middle age and later middle age unfortunately is often the time when either primary or secondary bone tumours can present. Primary tumours arise either within the bone or the dura and other intrinsic structures of the spinal canal, myeloma being probably the commonest form of lesion in bone. Secondary deposits arising from the breast, bronchus, ovary, thyroid and kidney are also common problems: we have seen secondary deposits 22 years plus after the removal of the primary lesion. With the advent of the large immigrant community in this country, osteomalacia has to be recognized as a cause of backache, as do infective causes, particularly tuberculosis. Finally, osteoporosis and osteoarthritis should not be overlooked as these can cause severe pain.

Table 7.1 *Common causes of backache*

Trauma
Mechanical back pain
Prolapsed intervertebral disc (PID)
Spina bifida
Sacro-ilitis
Infective
Tumour – primary and secondary
Osteoporosis and osteomalacia
Osteoarthritis
Sero-negative spondarthropathy
Paget's disease

HISTORY

A clear history should be sought of mode of onset of the back pain. Was the attack sudden or gradual? Does the pain stay in the same spot or does it move? Is there any radiation, particularly down a leg such as would be compatible with sciatica? (By definition sciatica is pain arising in the back, radiating into a buttock and going down a leg at least as far as the knee and possibly as far as the ankle. The pain is continuous in its distribution and may be severe.) Is there an associated arthritis? Have there been any fevers or night sweats? Have there been any skin or gut problems? Is the patient a recent immigrant, and has he any form of dietary restriction (polished rice or chappati on their own can lead to vitamin deficiency disease)? Has the patient indulged in any competitive sport or been involved in either a horseriding accident or trauma? It is worth remembering that a car accident in which a patient bangs his head or fractures his arm may also involve the back without the patient being aware of it. Is there any history of tumour? For example, if the patient has had a mastectomy or a lung resection then exclusion of a secondary deposit is essential. The key question in the history is whether or not the patient is kept awake by his symptoms; if this is the case and if the symptoms are getting worse this is generally of sinister import, and these are the patients who should be referred to hospital.

EXAMINATION

It is inadequate not to examine the patient with this condition properly; the patient should undress and be thoroughly examined. A careful observation of posture should be undertaken to look for a scoliosis or a kyphosis, as patients with prolapsed intervertebral disc often do have a scoliosis. Can the patient stand or does he find it difficult to do so? Is the lumbar lordosis increased or is there flattening of the spine? Flattening of the spine is found in association with ankylosing spondylitis. Increased lumbar lordosis may be a postural problem; this is encountered particularly in the West African community and can lead sometimes to quite marked ligament problems. Is the patient able to flex and extend his back? Rotation is also clearly important in the full examination. Examination of the back involves examination of the abdomen and of the breasts or testicles, i.e. a complete examination of the patient. Only at this point can investigations be considered.

49

Table 7.2 *Commoner causes of backache in various age groups*

Children	Scoliosis
	Spondylolisthesis
	Tumour
	TB in the spine
Adolescents	Spinal osteochondrosis
	(Scheuermann's disease)
	PID
	Mechanical
	Scoliosis
	Spondylolisthesis
	Spina bifida occulta
	TB in the spine
Young adults	PID
	Mechanical
	Ankylosing spondylitis
	TB
Middle-aged	PID
	Mechanical
	OA secondary to Scheuermann's and spondylolisthesis
	Paget's
	Coccydynia
	Spinal stenosis
Elderly	OA
	Osteoporosis
	Osteomalacia
	Metastases

INVESTIGATIONS

Investigations may be unnecessary. They are expensive and therefore should only be undertaken if a patient does not respond to rest. First investigations involve haemoglobin, a full blood count and ESR. It may be necessary to carry out a SMAC to include the plasma proteins, alkaline phosphatase, calcium and phosphate. This helps to include myeloma, underlying infection, secondary deposits, osteomalacia and osteoporosis (osteoporosis giving normal blood results, whereas in osteomalacia the alkaline phosphatase is invariably elevated). Another cause of raised alkaline phosphatase which may cause problems in differential diagnosis is a single Paget's vertebra.

X-rays may be helpful, showing degenerative disease or even collapse or crush fracture. In the presence of the possibility of infection or tumour, it may be necessary to undertake a bone biopsy in order to derive definite information. If the diagnosis is considered to be that of a prolapsed intervertebral disc, a myelogram (or a radiculogram) may be indicated. A myelogram is also indicated if there is a history suspicious of spinal canal stenosis – in this case the pain comes on when the patient walks and is relieved on resting but recurs when the patient walks again. This condition often produces sciatica as the root symptom.

TREATMENT

Patients with severe back pain should be confined to bed. Complete bed rest involves persuading the spouse that feeding should be confined to bed, that the patient should lie flat or in a comfortable position and that toilet and bath are the only reasons for moving from that posture. If the symptoms have not improved within 14 days, this is the sign for action.

There are signs which should alert the general practitioner to immediate action before thinking of bed rest. The presence of a neurological deficit, i.e. foot drop, paralysis of another myotome or a major deficit such as bowel or micturition problems, or extreme tenderness keeping the patient awake should alert the clinician to the underlying pathology being not mechanical but bony disease, and that this indicates the need for an urgent hospital opinion. This can either be obtained from the hospital casualty department or rheumatology outpatients department.

Mechanical backache will be relieved by a combination of analgesics and/or non-steroidal anti-inflammatory drugs and/or muscle relaxants. The secret is to aim for a high enough dose, for example paracetamol up to 4 grams daily, dihydrocodeine 30 mg 4 times daily, naproxen up to 1.5 grams daily, or valium up to

25 mg daily. If these measures fail, it suggests that there is underlying alternative pathology and even in the absence of neurological deficit a hospital referral is indicated.

The treatment of a prolapsed intervertebral disc is similar; failure of resolution should again indicate a hospital referral. Within a hospital environment, complete bed rest is again a reasonable approach. Some of these patients require traction, but there is no definite evidence that traction is in fact clinically effective in terms of relieving symptoms: all it achieves is that the patient remains in bed as he is immobilized by the pull. Failure to settle in a hospital ward is an indication for a myelogram and a neurosurgical referral with a view to decompression. There is an argument for the use of chemopapain but in the author's opinion, cases which are not too severe get better anyway, while very bad cases require surgery. Surgical decompression in the hands of a neurosurgeon or orthopaedic surgeon is sometimes indicated in the absence of improvement or with persistent severe neurological deficit. There are those who believe that early neurosurgical decompression is better than a conservative approach, but most would prefer the neurosurgical intervention only if the conservative approach failed. The argument for this is that the majority of disc problems are minor and settle with a conservative approach, and patients do not get recurrence of symptoms: for this reason we favour the conservative approach.

The treatment of ankylosing spondylitis and the associated sacro-iliac conditions is discussed further in Chapter 5 on sero-negative arthropathies. If infection is found in the spine, it is necessary to obtain the infective organism. A biopsy of an infective vertebra may well give this information. Treatment should only be given if one is sure of the organism.

PROGNOSIS

The prognosis for backache is extremely good. As stated at the beginning of this chapter, the majority of cases will settle. It is clearly important to pick out those with underlying disease, and the prognosis then depends on the disease one is treating. In the case of mechanical backache, whatever one does relieves symptoms – osteopathy, acupuncture, manipulative therapy or just simple bed rest. Alternative medicine is discussed in Chapter 14.

Table 7.3 *Functional distribution of lumbar and sacral roots*

Spinal root	Main muscles	Function	Main sensory distribution	Tendon reflexes
L3	Quadriceps	Knee extension	Front of knee	Knee
L4	Tibialis anterior	Foot dorsiflexion	Inner shin	Knee
L5	Extensor hallucis and digitorum longus	Toe dorsiflexion	Outer shin, dorsum or foot	—
S1	Gastrocnemius, soleus	Foot plantar flexion	Outer border of foot and sole	Ankle
S2, S3, S4	—	—	Perianal area and external genitalia	Cremasteric

8

Neck Pain

□ □ □ □ □ □ □ □ □ □ □ □

Although most people suffer from a painful neck at some stage during their life, most neck pain is benign and transient resolving within a few weeks with or without treatment.

PATHOPHYSIOLOGY

The mechanism of neck pain production is poorly understood. However, one view is that in young people the cause is frequently a herniating or ruptured intervertebral disc, and in older people it is the degenerative process which affects the same disc (i.e. cervical spondylosis). Another opinion is that a stiff painful neck in a young person is caused by a facet (synovial) joint dysfunction, and in the older patient it is again the degenerative changes which affect the same joints (i.e. osteoarthritis of facet joints). There are other pain-sensitive structures in and around the spine, e.g. paravertebral muscles and ligaments, from which neck pain can arise.

In addition to the above-described 'mechanical' pain, trauma and fibrositis can cause neck pain. But most importantly, a small number of more serious pathological causes (see Table 8.1) must be excluded.

Table 8.1 *Pathological causes of neck pain*

Tumours: cervical cord tumour, metastatic and primary tumour of the bone, multiple myeloma, lymphoma, metastatic tumour of lymph nodes, soft tissue tumour (carotid and thyroid)

Meningitis and meningism

Soft tissue cysts (e.g. branchial and thyroglossal)

Sub-acute thyroiditis

Inflammatory arthropathies (e.g. rheumatoid arthritis, chronic juvenile arthritis, the spondarthropathies)

Polymyalgia rheumatica/giant cell arthritis

Dental causes

Psychogenic neck pain is rare and the diagnosis must never be made unless there are positive psychogenic signs and malignancy and infection in the bone have been carefully excluded. Most of the conditions which cause neck pain may cause shoulder pain at the same time; at times the shoulder pain may be predominant.

Table 8.2 *Causes of neck pain*

Traumatic

Mechanical

Pathological

Fibrositis

PRESENTATIONS

Neck pain may present in one of six main syndromes (Table 8.3).

56

Table 8.3 *Presentation of neck pain*

Syndrome	Cause	Onset	Severity of pain	Stiffness
Whiplash injury	Trauma	Sudden	Very severe	Neck held in one position
Torticollis (acute wryneck)	PID/facet dysfunction	Acute (hours)	Severe	Neck held in one position of rest
Neck pain and/or arm pain (root compression)	PID	Acute or sub-acute (usually days)	Severe	One or two movements limited and painful
Cervical spondylosis	Degenerative changes in discs and facet joints	Chronic (months or years)	Variable; generally less severe	Lateral flexion and rotation mainly affected
Malignant neck pain	Infection or neoplasm of bone	Sudden or gradual	Very severe; unremitting even when immobile. Night pain with tenderness over several vertebrae	Pain is present in any position of movement or rest. True stiffness is lacking
Fibrositis	Inadequate non-REM sleep	Gradual	Variable; accompanied by tender points in various areas (lateral epicondyles, trapezius, supraspinatus, lower cervical spine, lower lumbar spine, gluteus medius, medial fat pads on thighs)	Variable; generally less severe

57

1. Whiplash injury

It is a necessary coincidence that whiplash injury has become more common since the introduction of the compulsory wearing of front seat belts; this is partly due to the lack of adequate back head rests. Persistent neck pain with or without root signs may also follow road traffic accidents, a fall from a height of over four metres, gymnastics, rugby, etc. The pain is usually around the C6–7 and TI–2 vertebrae: bone injury at the latter site may require lateral computerized tomography for its demonstration.

Less severe injury may precipitate or aggravate neck pain due to pre-existing cervical spondylosis, and this may be significant if there is a compensation claim.

X-rays should be taken in flexion and extension to detect unstable fracture/dislocation, as well as special views for the odontoid peg.

2. Torticollis (acute wryneck)

This often affects young people. The patient usually wakes up one morning with a stiff neck with the head tilted to one side. The muscle affected is usually the sternocleidomastoid but the trapezius or other such muscles may be the cause. The pain is very severe and the neck is held in one position to avoid aggravation of the pain. The condition is transient and usually resolves within a week or two; it is thought to be caused by facet joint dysfunction or a prolapsed intervertebral disc.

Torticollis should not be confused with 'spasmodic torticollis' which is a form of focal torsion dystonia beginning in adulthood and remaining limited to the affected part of the body. It tends to be persistent and can be painful.

3. Acute protrusion or rupture of cervical intervertebral disc

This can occur at any age. Although the severe pain and stiffness usually occurs suddenly, it may well be mild at first but increase in severity over a period of days and sometimes even weeks. In severe cases the pain is referred to the dermatome of one of the cervical nerve roots and may be accompanied with tingling in very severe cases. One or more of the muscles supplied by the compressed root may be weak, and the appropriate tendon reflex may be diminished or even absent (see Table 8.4). The neck is usually very stiff and one or two movements are very limited and painful, certain movements may aggravate arm pain as well as parasthaesia.

Most cases will resolve within a few weeks, but patients with neurological signs take longer to recover and in some cases the recovery may never be complete.

4. Cervical spondylosis

The term cervical spondylosis is usually reserved for the degenerative changes affecting the cervical discs whereas the term osteoarthritis is used to describe the degenerative changes in the facet joints. Cervical spondylosis affects 90% of men over the age of 50 and 90% of women over the age of 60, but very few patients become symptomatic. Of these, the symptoms merely consist of pain and/or stiffness in the neck of variable severity, but generally less severe than in the conditions described previously. The condition usually develops gradually over months or even years, and a number of patients may have root signs (see Table 8.4).

Table 8.4 *Functional distribution of cervical nerve roots*

Spinal roots	Main muscles	Function	Main sensory distribution	Tendon reflexes
C2			Posterior half of head, upper half of neck	
C3	Trapezius	Shoulder shrugging	Lower half of neck	
C4	Trapezius	Shoulder shrugging	Supraclavicular fossae, front of chest below clavicles	
C5	Deltoid biceps, brachialis	Elbow flexion Shoulder abduction	Anterolateral shoulder	Biceps
C6	Extensor carpi radialis	Wrist extension	Thumb	Supinator
C7	Triceps	Elbow extension	Middle finger	Triceps
C8	Flexor digitoum	Finger flexion	Little finger	
T1	Hand	Abduction and adduction of fingers	Medial arm	

Some patients, especially those with a narrow cervical canal, may present with upper motor neurone weakness of one or both legs; this is followed over months or years by weakness in the upper limbs. The spinothalamic tracts may be involved as well, causing loss of pain and temperature sensation in the lower limbs, and in some cases proprioception (dorsal column) may also be affected. Sensory involvement in the upper limbs is usually of a dermatomal pattern. This condition is thought to occur in patients with a congenitally narrowed cervical canal. The spinal cord has a diameter of 9–10 mm and if the anterior–posterior diameter of the spinal canal is 10 mm or less, the patient is more liable to suffer cord compression with posterior herniation of the degenerated discs: however, the neck symptoms and signs are usually minimal.

The vertebral arteries which pass through the transverse foramina of the cervical vertebrae may be compressed by osteophytes thus leading to sudden drop attacks or vertigo, especially following sudden twisting movements of the neck.

Table 8.5 *Presentation of cervical spondylosis*

Asymptomatic
Localized pain and/or stiffness
Root pressure (radiculopathy)
Cord compression (cervical spondylotic myelopathy)
Brain stem ischaemia (vertebro-basilar insufficiency)

5. Malignant neck pain

Although this is uncommon, it should always be excluded when the patient develops sudden and severe pain in the cervical spine. The pain is usually continuous and unremitting even when the patient is resting and the neck is immobile. Night pain is very severe and is accompanied by tenderness over several vertebrae. True stiffness is lacking and the patient has great difficulty in finding a position of rest. A neoplasm should always be excluded, especially secondary: osteomyelitis is the other possibility. Suspicion of a neoplasm or infection is perhaps the main indication for sending a patient with neck pain and without a history of preceding trauma for cervical X-rays. In some cases the X-rays are normal, in which case a bone scan might be helpful.

6. Fibrositis (see Chapter 10)

This is a common cause of mild to severe niggly pain at the back of the neck and in the trapezius muscles. Although the onset is usually gradual, it is sometimes sudden and may follow mechanical neck or back pain. The condition is usually accompanied by tender points (trigger spots) in various areas (the lateral epicondyles, trapezius, supraspinatus, lower cervical spine, lower lumbar spine, gluteus medius, medial fat pads of the thighs) which are unknown to the patient but are discovered on physical examination.

Fibrositis is thought to be due to inadequate non-rapid eye movement sleep. There might be some limitation of cervical movement but root symptoms and signs are lacking. Tricyclic antidepressants are more useful than diazepam in ensuring a good night's sleep. There are other controversial methods of treatment.

MANAGEMENT OF MECHANICAL NECK PAIN

The nature of the neck pain must be explained thoroughly and the patient must be reassured about the nature of his symptoms. The ARC booklet on neck pain is very useful.

It is generally agreed on no known scientific grounds that a properly fitting soft collar is useful in alleviating the pain. The collar can be worn even at night. For more severe cases, especially with root symptoms and signs, a firm collar can be worn, and in severe cases admission to hospital and continuous cervical traction might be needed. Simple non-narcotic analgesics are useful in alleviating the pain, and in more severe cases codeine or dihydrocodeine and/or a non-steroidal anti-inflammatory drug might be of help. The patient should also be advised to use a low pillow.

Once the pain subsides and some movement is possible, exercises should be encouraged and the patient should practice forward flexion, backward flexion, lateral and rotational movement. The exercises should be continued regularly even after the pain has completely subsided.

There is some evidence that manipulation of the neck by an osteopath or physiotherapist experienced in neck problems may be curative in patients with acute wryneck, but under no circumstances should the neck be manipulated if there are any symptoms or signs of root compression as this can aggravate the problem. Manipulation should never be performed without X-rays of the cervical spine.

In patients with severe chronic pain arising from spondylosis, transcutaneous nerve stimulation might be of help, and before the patient is asked to buy or rent his own machine it should be demonstrated in a physiotherapy department that application of the TNS machine over a period of 1–2 hours does alleviate the pain. There is also some evidence that acupuncture is helpful to some patients, more so than in treatment of low backache.

Most patients with neck pain can be managed by their general practitioner. The following patients should be referred to the hospital:

(1)   The patient with severe neck pain especially when it is not relieved within a few days with the above measures.

(2)   Where malignancy or infection of bone is suspected.

(3)   The patient with neurological signs.

(4)   When the general practitioner is unsure of the diagnosis.

Table 8.6 *Treatment of mechanical neck pain*

Explanation and reassurance
Rest: total and/or local
Analgesia
Palliative physiotherapy (heat, ice, ultrasound, etc.)
Hour-glass pillow
Collars
Neck exercises
Traction (continuous or intermittent)
Manipulation
Alternative medicine (TNS, acupuncture)
Surgery

9

The Painful Shoulder

☐ ☐ ☐ ☐ ☐ ☐ ☐ ☐ ☐ ☐ ☐ ☐ ☐

Of prime importance is the recognition that pain felt in the shoulder may be referred from disorders of the cervical spine, lungs, pleura, heart, pericardium, diaphragm and even sub-diaphragmatic areas. Cervical spondylosis is perhaps the commonest cause of shoulder pain. Median nerve compression at the wrist may also be a cause. Other causes include secondary and primary bone diseases and systemic conditions like polymyalgia rheumatica and rheumatoid arthritis. After the above causes have been excluded, there remains a group of painful disorders which affect the muscles and the periarticular soft tissues around the three independent articulations of the shoulder complex: the glenohumeral, acromioclavicular and sternoclavicular joints as well as the scapulo-thoracic joints. The latter conditions are described briefly in this chapter.

ADHESIVE CAPSULITIS (FROZEN SHOULDER)

The main two features of this condition are pain and limitation of movement in the shoulder. Typically, it starts with pain in the shoulder which increases in severity within a few days and becomes persistent throughout the day and night. At the same time, there is a progressive loss of both active and passive movements at the shoulder. The first movement to be lost is external rotation which may later become extremely restricted; abduction and internal rotation are affected to a lesser degree. In some cases there might be complete loss of all glenohumeral movements and all the movement that is possible in the shoulder is mainly scapulothoracic. The condition is usually self-limiting, the pain subsiding within a few weeks to a few months. The restriction of movements takes longer to disappear – up to two years – and may never be complete.

The cause of adhesive capsulitis remains obscure, but it is commoner after the age of forty and its peak incidence is between the ages of fifty and seventy, being perhaps slightly commoner in women than in men. Although most cases of frozen shoulder develop spontaneously, the following patients have a higher risk:

1. Stroke patients.

2. Diabetics, possibly due to increased glucosylation of the collagen fibres.

3. Parkinson's disease.

4. Herpes zoster.

5. Patients who have undergone thoracic surgery for breast cancer.

In this group of patients prevention is important; early mobilization and active movement of the shoulder is of paramount importance.

Pathologically, the tightened thickened capsule of the shoulder is responsible for the limitation of movement and histologically it shows fibrosis and reparative inflammatory changes.

Early institution of mobilizing exercises is perhaps most successful in halting the progression of shoulder immobility. An injection of corticosteroid into the glenohumeral joint may help ease the pain. In resistant cases, manipulation under general anaesthesia followed by intensive mobilizing physiotherapy may be indicated.

ACROMIOCLAVICULAR JOINT STRAIN

The pain in this condition is usually felt over the tip of the shoulder and arises mainly on movement of the arm above the level of the shoulder. Physical examination usually reveals tenderness over the acromioclavicular joint and the pain is reproduced in the extreme few degrees of abduction and in internal rotation. This condition is not uncommon in a sportsman. It responds rapidly to a local corticosteroid injection into the acromioclavicular joint. Very rarely, persistent cases end up in acromionectomy.

CALCIFIC PERIARTHRITIS (CALCIFYING SUPRASPINATUS TENDINITIS)

This is a form of soft tissue psuedogout and is caused by the local deposition of calcium salt in and around the supraspinatus tendon. Sometimes these deposits evoke a severe inflammatory reaction causing sudden severe incapacitating pain. The shoulders become acutely tender and often swollen and warm to the touch. Infection is usually suspected but an X-ray of the shoulder will show calcium deposits. It is treated with a local steroid injection with anaesthetic and a non-steroidal anti-inflammatory drug is often prescribed to help in reducing the inflammation. The patient will start to feel better within a few hours of the injection, and within a few days most symptoms will disappear. Some orthopaedic surgeons might attempt to aspirate the pasty calcium salts under general anaesthesia. The calcium deposits may persist but surgical removal is rarely necessary as a follow-up X-ray will show that they have shrunk in size or even disappeared.

NEURALGIC AMYOTROPHY

Neuralgic amyotrophy is another cause of acute, severe shoulder pain. Typically, it starts with aching pain felt around the shoulder or less often around the elbow and forearm. However, muscle weakness develops within a few hours or days; sensory loss is usually minimal. In mild cases, improvement is within a few weeks and the clinical recovery is complete within a few months, but more often in severe cases improvement does not begin for several months and may not be complete for a few years. Nevertheless, eventual or almost complete recovery is likely. Nerve-conduction studies might reveal more extensive involvement of the nerves than expected from the clinical examination. The cerebrospinal fluid is usually normal and apart from adequate pain relief and mobilizing physiotherapy to prevent stiffening of the shoulder, there is no known treatment.

BICIPITAL TENDONITIS

The pain in this condition frequently radiates along the biceps to the forearm. Tenderness is localized over the bicipital groove of the humerus where the tendon lies. The pain is usually aggravated by abduction and internal rotation and is also accentuated with resisted supination of the forearm with the elbow flexed at 90°.

Bicipital tendonitis responds promptly to a local corticosteroid injection. Pathologically there is inflammation and degeneration of the long head of the biceps and sometimes the changes are so severe that they may lead to a rupture of the tendon which would appear like a ping-pong ball in the bulk of the biceps muscle. The treatment in such cases is mainly conservative, and surgical exploration with tendon transfer is rarely needed.

THE PAINFUL ARC SYNDROME

The tendons of the subscapularis, suprasinatus, infraspinatus and teres minor muscles are all intermittently blended with the fibrous capsule of the shoulder joint forming a cuff sometimes termed the rotator cuff; they reinforce the capsule and hence provide active support for the joint during movement, and because they are all inserted to the upper end of the humerus, they function much of the time to retain the head of the humerus in its correct alignment relative to the glenoid cavity. The tendons of these muscles may suffer degenerative changes, hence giving rise to pain in the shoulder with certain movements. Examination usually reveals full passive and active movement, but there is pain on abduction with the palm facing the floor between 45° and 120°. The commonest of these tendons to be affected is the supraspinatus where the tenderness is just anterior to the acromioclavicular joint and the pain can be reproduced on resisted abduction of the arm. When the infraspinatus and the teres minor are involved, the tenderness is usually posterior to the acromioclavicular joint and the pain can be reproduced on resisted external rotation. Rarely, the tendon of the subscapularis may be affected giving tenderness in front of the shoulder and pain which is reproduced on resisted internal rotation.

These conditions respond promptly to a local steroid injection and the response is more prolonged if the injection is done at the anatomical position of the tendons rather than at the tender spot.

Sometimes the patient has a painful arm, but all the resisted movements are pain-free. This arises when there is inflammation of the subacromial bursa and it also responds to a local steroid injection. The needle is placed in the gap between the acromioclavicular arch and the head of the humerus with the needle going horizontally but slightly tilted in a superior direction.

OSTEOARTHRITIS OF THE SHOULDER

Osteoarthritis of the shoulder is not uncommon, but a previous history of trauma might be elicited from some patients. Both shoulders can be affected with symptoms much less pronounced than in the above-described conditions, and the patient gives a long history of increasing pain with some limitation of almost all the movements of the shoulder. Loud crepitus may be present. This condition shares similar features with adhesive capsulitis, but they are never as pronounced as in the latter. Most patients would be satisfied with a careful explanation of the nature of this noncrippling condition. Local corticosteroid injection is not indicated and physiotherapy rarely helps, but simple analgesics or non-steroidal anti-inflammatory drugs may help to ease the pain.

THE SHOULDER–HAND SYNDROME

This condition usually presents with pain and stiffness in the shoulder together with pain, swelling and vasomotor phenomena in the hands later in the disease. The changes in the hands may resemble those of Sudeck's atrophy, and the shoulder may become 'frozen'. This syndrome is poorly understood, but it principally affects patients over the age of 50 and is often associated with an acute illness such as myocardial infarction trauma, stroke or pulmonary disease.

Aggressive phsyiotherapy is more important here than in any other shoulder condition. In severe cases stellate ganglion block or regional infusion with guanethidine may be tried.

Table 9.1 *Management of the painful shoulder*

Syndrome	Shoulder pain	Painful arc	Pain on resisted movement	Limitation of movement	Treatment
Adhesive capsulitis	Diffuse	—	—	All movements markedly limited	Mobilization + IA steroid
Acromioclavicular joint strain	At tip of shoulder	120° – 150°	—	—	Local steroid into AC joint
Calcific periarthritis	Severe and diffuse	—	—	All movement limited.	Local steroid + NSAI
Neuralgic amyotrophy	Severe and diffuse	—	—	Passive movements full	Analgesics + mobility
Bicipital tendinitis	Localized	—	Elbow flexion Wrist supination	—	Local steroid
Subacromial bursitis	Localized	45° – 120°	—	—	Local steroid
Supraspinatous tendinitis	Localized	45° – 120°	Abduction	—	Local steroid
Infraspinatus tendinitis	Localized	45° – 120°	External rotation	—	Local steroid
Subscapularis tendinitis	Localized	45° – 120°	Internal rotation	—	Local steroid
Osteoarthritis of shoulder	Long history, increasing diffuse	—	—	Some limitation of all movement	Explanation + analgesics + NSAI
Infection	Severe and diffuse	—	—	All movements limited by pain	Refer to hospital: drainage + antibiotics + analgesics

10

Soft Tissue Rheumatism

☐ ☐ ☐ ☐ ☐ ☐ ☐ ☐ ☐ ☐ ☐ ☐ ☐

The conditions described in this chapter are mostly caused by simple non-serious disease affecting tendons, tendinous attachment to bone, supporting collagen tissue and entrapped peripheral nerves. Most of them require simple treatment (e.g. local steroid injection or proper splinting) and explanation to the patient of the benign nature of the condition.

TRIGGER FINGER AND THUMB

The flexor tendons of the fingers move smoothly inside a covering fibrous sheath. Thickening or nodule formation in either the tendon or its fibrous sheath can lead to triggering: when the fingers are extended, the affected finger lags behind and then suddenly straightens itself out with or without help. The middle and ring fingers are most commonly affected. The thickening or the nodule is usually palpable opposite the metacarpo-phalangeal joint. Injecting around the thickening or the nodule with local steroid generally leads to a quick cure; otherwise surgical division of the tendon sheath at the level of the metacarpo-phalangeal joint ensures an immediate cure.

DEQUERVAIN'S TENOSYNOVITIS

Tenosynovitis of the extensor pollicis brevis and abductor pollicis longus causes pain and tenderness over the radial side of the wrist. The condition is commonly subacute or chronic and is aggravated by excessive repetitive use of the hands as in gardening and knitting.

Careful examination reveals swelling over the radial styloid. The Finkelstein test is positive: the patient is asked to make a fist with the thumb folded into the palm and the remaining fingers flexed over it. The examiner gently deviates the fist to the ulnar side, thus putting the inflamed tendon on the stretch resulting in sudden exacerbation of the pain.

Local steroid injection with 1% lignocaine in the tendon sheath leads to rapid relief of the pain.

ENTRAPMENT NEUROPATHIES

The peripheral nerves may be compressed at various levels during their course giving rise to pain, parasthaesia and weakness distal to the site of the lesion. The entrapment neuropathies are summarized in Table 10.1. The commonest of these neuropathies is the carpal tunnel syndrome discussed below.

Table 10.1 *Some of the common entrapment neuropathies*

Syndrome	Nerve involved	Site of pressure	Main symptoms and signs
Saturday night palsy	Radial	Axilla	Wrist drop
Posterior interosseous nerve compression	Posterior interosseous	Supinater	Weakness of finger and thumb extension
Ulnar tunnel	Ulnar	Behind medial epicondyle	Pain on medial side of forearm and pain and loss of sensation of IV and V fingers
Ulnar carpal tunnel	Ulnar	Between pisiform and hook of hamate	Weakness of intrinsic muscles and loss of sensation of IV and V fingers
Anterior interosseous nerve compression	Anterior interosseous	Fibrous origin of flexor digitorum sublimis	Weakness of flexion of thumb, index and middle fingers
Carpal tunnel	Median	Under flexor retinaculum	Pain, parasthaesia and impaired sensation of thumb, index and middle fingers
Meralgia parasthetica	Lateral cutaneous nerve of thigh	Medial to anterior supine iliac spine	Pain and impaired sensation on lateral aspect of thigh
Common peroneal nerve compression	Common peroneal	Fibular neck	Pain on shin and dorsum of foot with foot drop
Tarsal tunnel	Posterior tibial	Flexor retinaculum	Pain and parasthesia on sole of foot

Carpal tunnel syndrome

The median nerve may be compressed under the flexor retinaculum in the carpal tunnel at the wrist. This commonly occurs as an isolated condition or may rarely be secondary to other conditions such as rheumatoid arthritis, pregnancy, myxoedema, acromegaly, diabetes mellitus, Colles' fracture and fracture of the scaphoid bone.

The patient usually presents with severe pain in the hand especially during the night. Often the patient has to shake his hands several times for a few minutes before the pain subsides. The pain may radiate to the elbows and even to the shoulder and is often accompanied by paraesthesiae over the thumb, index and middle fingers. In severe cases the patient notices weakness in holding a pen or book between the thumb and index fingers. Examination often confirms diminished or lost sensation over the thumb and lateral two fingers, and weakness of thumb abduction. Tapping the median nerve at the wrist causes a shock of pain in the fingers (Tinel's sign). In severe cases there is wasting of the thenar muscles. The diagnosis is confirmed by demonstrating delayed conduction of the median nerve at the wrist.

In mild cases the pain may be relieved by wearing a resting wrist splint, especially at night. A short-acting diuretic may also help by reducing the oedema at the wrist. A local steroid injection (between the flexor carpi radialis and palmaris longus at the distal wrist crease) may only rarely help severe cases. Resistant cases may need surgical release of the flexor retinaculum; thenar wasting is an absolute indication for surgery.

THE ENTHESOPATHIES

The term enthesopathy is used to describe painful conditions characterized by inflammation at the site of attachment of tendons and ligaments to bone.

Table 10.3 *The enthesopathies*

Site of pain and tenderness	Syndrome
Heel	Plantar fasciitis
Achilles tendon	Achilles tendonitis
Iliac crest	—
Ischial tuberosity	—
Lateral epicondyle	Tennis elbow
Medial epicondyle	Golfer's elbow

Plantar fasciitis, Achilles tendonitis, pain and tenderness over the iliac crest and ischial tuberosity are often associated with HLA-B27 spondarthritis (ankylosing spondylitis, etc.). These conditions are discussed in Chapter 11 on foot pain.

Tennis elbow (lateral epicondylitis) and golfer's elbow (medial epicondylitis)

These two conditions are usually caused by repetitive movements involving the long extensors of the hands and fingers (lateral epicondylitis) or the long flexors of the hands and fingers (medial epicondylitis); they are therefore not only precipitated by playing tennis or golf but by decorating, book binding, window cleaning, etc. The patient usually complains of pain at the elbow radiating to the hand especially when using the appropriate muscles. The tenderness is about $\frac{1}{2}$–1 cm distal to the lateral or medial epicondyle. The pain can be produced by flexing the elbow and forcefully resisting dorsiflexion (tennis elbow) or flexion (golfer's elbow) of the forcefully closed fist.

In most patients, this condition is self-limiting. In more severe cases a local steroid injection with 1% lignocaine is effective in relieving the pain, and the injection may be repeated. Local ultrasound therapy is sometimes helpful but time-consuming. An elbow band may be worn over the elbow or upper part of the forearm.

The patient should be taught to avoid using his hands with the forearm in supination in the case of tennis elbow or pronation in the case of golfer's elbow and to use the hand with the forearm in the opposite position. Severe resistant cases may require immobilization of the elbow in Baycast or POP for 3–4 weeks. Surgery is rarely required.

BURSITIS

There are over 150 bursae distributed in the body and any of these can become inflamed and painful. Repeated trauma is the commonest cause and certain occupations predispose to the formation of inflamed bursae; examples are Olcranon bursitis (miner's elbow, student elbow, drunkard's elbow), ischial bursitis (weaver's bottom) and prepatellar bursitis (clergyman's knee, nun's knee, housemaid's knee, carpet layer's knee). The presentation may be sudden and acute or symptomless and chronic. Other more important causes are infection and the presence of urate crystals. Bursitis is also commonly found in association with inflammatory arthritis especially rheumatoid arthritis.

Because of the fear of infection, inflamed bursae must be aspirated and the fluid examined for crystals as well as cultured bacteriologically including special cultures for *Mycobacterium tuberculosis*. Aspiration leads to rapid pain relief and if infection is excluded a local steroid injection will accelerate cure. Chronic and recurrently inflamed bursae may have to be excised.

Trochanteric bursitis (over the greater trochanter) deserves a special mention. This may be confused with arthritis of the hip joint; eliciting local tenderness by pressure on the greater trochanter proves the diagnosis. A local steroid injection is usually symptomatically effective.

Bursitis on the medial side of the knee is associated with osteoarthritis of the knee. The pain and tenderness is localized to the medial aspect of the knee, and is worse at night. The pain is usually more severe than that caused by uncomplicated osteoarthritis. A local steroid injection leads to rapid pain relief.

HYPERMOBILITY SYNDROME

Hypermobility or lax joints should always be considered when a young or middle-aged person complains of vague aches and pains which may or may not be related to the joints, especially the knees, hands and lower lumbar spine. The pain is usually aggravated by trauma. The condition may be secondary to some genetic diseases, e.g. osteogenesis imperfecta, Ehlers–Danlos syndrome, Marfan's syndrome and homocystinuria. It may also be associated with Turner's syndrome and Down's syndrome, but more commonly it occurs without evidence of an underlying disease but may be associated with varicose veins and a prolapsed mitral valve. It is usually familial. Hypermobility is normal in the early years of life and in gymnasts and ballet dancers.

To diagnose this condition hypermobility needs to be demonstrated by the following manoeuvres:

1. Hyperextending both little fingers to 90°.

2. Touching the radial aspect of the forearm with the thumb (on each side).

3. Hyperextending both elbows by more than 10°.

4. Hyperextending both knees by more than 10°.

5. Placing the hands flat on the floor while standing with the knees straight.

There is no specific treatment for this condition but reassuring the patient is important. Most patients would be relieved to know that there is an explanation for their complaints and that they are not imagining their symptoms.

Patients with hypermobile joints tend to develop degenerative joint changes earlier than normal.

FIBROSITIS

The term fibrositis (a misnomer) is used to describe a syndrome where trunk or limb pain is accompanied by tenderness over several trigger points (of which the patient is usually unaware) but without other objective signs. The cause is unknown but it is thought that inadequate deep sleep (non-rapid eye movement sleep) may be an important aetiological factor. Fibrositis may complicate a painful neck or low backache due to other causes.

Physical examination shows consistent trigger or tender spots. It is suggested that there are 14 of these which are well defined: on the trapezius (right and left), second costo-chondral junction (right and left), 1–2 cm distal to the lateral epicondyles on both sides, supraspinatus (right and left), lower cervical and lumbar spine, gluteus medius (right and left) and medial fat pad of the lower part of the thigh (right and left).

Treatment starts with reassurance and explanation to the patient of the benign nature of the condition. Tricyclic antidepressants (e.g. imipramine or trimipramine 75 mg nocte) are effective in ensuring a good night's sleep and this may produce dramatic relief. Use of a soft collar at night, heat therapy, massage and transcutaneous nerve stimulation (TNS) are also helpful.

11

The Painful Foot

☐ ☐ ☐ ☐ ☐ ☐ ☐ ☐ ☐ ☐ ☐ ☐

Ill-fitting footwear is perhaps the biggest single cause of a painful foot. Children and teenagers should be encouraged to participate in barefoot activities and in the wearing of well-fitting sandals. They should be discouraged from wearing fashion shoes with excessively high heels and pointed toes. The best footwear is perhaps the type which allows the foot to be held well into the heel of the shoe and allows the toes to move freely upwards and downwards and from side to side. Female fashion shoes are responsible for most cases of hallux valgus, hammer toe deformities, painful callosities and flexed and over-ridden small toes. Most adult British women suffer from hallux valgus, and although in about half of them there is a familial predisposition, ill-fitting footwear contributes to this high incidence. Non-porous sports shoes also contribute to the incidence of athletes foot, other skin infections and ingrowing toe nails.

The diagnosis and management of the painful foot has been subdivided into three parts for the sake of simplicity and is summarized in Tables 11.1, 11.2 and 11.3. The division of the foot into fore-, mid- and hindfoot is arbitrary: the forefoot is anterior to the tarsus, the hindfoot is the area of the calcaneus and talsus and the midfoot is the rest of the tarsal bones. In this chapter some of the more common conditions will be discussed in detail.

Table 11.1 *Management of forefoot pain*

Site of pain and/or tenderness	Syndrome	Treatment
2nd or 3rd metatarsal shaft	March (stress) fracture	Walking POP or Baycast for 6 weeks
2nd metatarsal head	Freiberg's disease	Rest or ignore
Intermetatarsal spaces especially 3rd and 4th	Neuroma	Surgery
1st MTP joint	(a) Gout	Indocid or colchicine
	(b) Hallux rigidus (OA)	Pad; analgesics; injection; surgery
	(c) Hallux valgus (bunion)	Pad; inject bunion; surgery
Head of 5th metatarsal	Bunionette	Pad; inject bunion; surgery
2nd or 3rd cleft	Morton's metatarsalgia	Surgery
MTP and PIP	Rheumatoid arthritis	NSAID and rocker-bar
DIP	Sero-negative arthritis	NSAID
3rd or 4th toe	'Sausage toe' (seronegative arthritis)	NSAID
Sole of foot	(a) Plantar warts	Caustics or cryosurgery Chiropody
	(b) Callosities and corns	

Table 11.2 *Management of midfoot pain*

Site of pain and/or tenderness	Syndrome	Treatment
Arch	Pes planus	Insole and intrinsic muscle exercises
Navicular	Köhler's disease	Rest or ignore
Dorsum	(a) Extensor tenosynovitis	Local steroid injection; ultrasound
	(b) Midtarsal strain	Rest and NSAID

Table 11.3 *Management of hindfoot pain*

Site of pain and/or tenderness	Syndrome	Treatment
Achilles tendon	Achilles tendonitis	Rest; ultrasound; stretching exercises
Lower end of achilles tendon	Sub-Achilles bursitis	Local steroid injection avoiding TA
Anterior to achilles tendon	Ante-Achilles bursitis	Local steroid injection
Back of calcaneum	Sever's disease	Rest or ignore
Heel	Plantar fasciitis	Local steroid injection; sorbo rubber heel pad
Behind and below medial malleolus	(a) Flexor tenosynovitis	Local steroid injection or ulstrasound
	(b) Medial ligament strain	Rest or NSAID or local steroid injection
Behind and below lateral malleolus	(a) Peroneal tenosynovitis	Local steroid injection and/or ultrasound
	(b) Lateral ligament strain	Rest or NSAID or local steroid injection

FLAT FOOT (PES PLANUS)

Flat feet are so common that it is important to remember that they may not be the cause of the patient's pain. Pain-free flat feet require no treatment; if flat feet do cause pain it is usually due to overstretching of the muscles and ligaments of the foot accentuated by obesity and occupational factors. Continuous overstretching of the soft tissue leads to forefoot hyperpronation and valgus deformity of the heel.

Flat feet may be flaccid, spastic or rigid. Most flat feet are flaccid, the longitudinal arch becoming depressed only in weight bearing. Spastic flat feet result from peroneal muscle spasm, hence inversion is limited and painful. When contracture develops, the foot becomes fixed in abduction which is why this condition is called rigid flat foot.

Keen long-distance runners with flat feet may suffer from knee pain due to the altered mechanics of the lower limbs. These patients and those with foot strain may benefit from wearing an insole which maintains the longitudinal arch; this relieves not only the foot pain but also the knee pain. Foot exercises should be encouraged to prevent progression of the flaccid flat foot to spastic and rigid flat foot.

PES CAVUS

This condition is the opposite to flat feet, i.e. over-accentuation of the longitudinal arch associated with clawing of the toes. If pes cavus causes pain it is usually due to painful callosities under the metatarsal heads; hammer toes with painful corns may also result. Later in adult life degenerative changes start in the tarsus as well as the toes causing more pain and disability. Although most cases are asymptomatic when first discovered, the patient should be advised to have built-in metatarsal supports in his shoes. Foot exercises are also to be encouraged. Some cases of pes cavus are associated with peroneal muscular atropathy (Charcot–Marie–Tooth syndrome), Friedreich's ataxia, spastic diplegia and old poliomyelitis, but in most cases no other features are found, although it is believed that these patients may represent the mild cases of peroneal muscular dystrophy.

JUVENILE OSTEOCHONDRITIS (OSTEOCHONDROSES)

Osteochondritis affects children and teenagers. There are three types which cause painful feet:

(1) Sever's disease affects mainly 6–10 year-old children and is caused by osteochondritis of the posterior apophysis of the calcaneus at the attachment of the tendo achilles. The pain and tenderness are localized to the insertion of the tendo achilles.

(2) Köhler's disease affects mainly 3–10 year-old children and is due to osteochondritis (or more correctly osteonecrosis) of

the navicular bone. The pain and tenderness are localized to the medial side of the midfoot.

(3) Freiberg's disease affects mainly 12–16 year-old children and is caused by osteochondritis of the epiphyseal centre of the second metatarsal bone. The pain and tenderness are localized to the forefoot and wriggling of the second metatarsal provokes severe tenderness.

These three conditions are self-limiting and settle down without any treatment within a few months. If the pain is severe, and supporting padding and insoles do not help, then putting the foot in Baycast or walking POP for a few weeks will relieve the pain.

HALLUX RIGIDUS

This is osteoarthritis of the first metatarso-phalangeal (MTP) joint. The onset is gradual with pain and stiffness on walking. Simple analgesics (paracetamol, aspirin or benorylate solution) may help, and a rocker-bar incorporated in the shoe under the MTP joint may ease the pain. If the pain is disabling, severe arthroplasty is then indicated.

HAMMER TOE AND MALLET TOE

Hammer toe is caused by fixed flexion deformity at the proximal interphalangeal joint of the big toe with compensatory hyperextension of the terminal joint. A mallet toe is a dropped terminal phalanx of the toe caused by rupture of the extensor tendons.

These two conditions cause pain due to the formation of callosities. Wider well-padded shoes may ease the pain, otherwise surgery is indicated.

ACHILLES TENDONITIS

This usually follows unaccustomed walking or jogging. The affected tendon may be thickened and is usually very tender at one spot. Achilles tendonitis should be differentiated from bursitis where the tenderness would be anterior to the tendon; this is important from the treatment point of view as the bursa may be injected but the tendon should not as it may rupture. Perhaps the local injection is best carried out in a hospital environment.

This condition is perhaps best treated by rest and local ultrasound therapy, and stretching exercises are also helpful. In severe cases the foot may have to be immobilized in walking POP or Baycast.

Achilles tendonitis may be a marker for seronegative arthritis (ankylosing spondylitis, Reiter's syndrome, colitic and psoriatic spondarthritis), and it is therefore important to examine for tenderness in the sacro-iliac joints and restriction of movements in the spine and chest expansion.

PLANTAR FASCIITIS

This condition causes pain and tenderness in the heel. X-rays may show a calcaneal spur but this is unlikely to be the cause as spurs are common and rarely give rise to any heel pain. Plantar fasciitis may occur in the absence of a spur. Local steroid injection with 1% lignocaine relieves the pain; it is less painful to introduce the needle from the medial side of the heel rather than from the sole. A sorbo rubber heel pad is also helpful.

Plantar fasciitis, like Achilles tendonitis, may also be a marker for seronegative arthritis. X-rays in these cases may show a fluffy spur with erosions.

GOUT

Gouty arthritis (monosodium urate monohydrate crystal

synovitis) commonly presents with sudden severe pain, swelling and redness of the first metatarso-phalangeal joint of the big toe in a middle-aged man. The local tenderness is usually exquisite. The patient may be feverish, and there may be moderate leukocytosis. In the early days the X-ray is usually normal apart from soft tissue swelling: after repeated attacks erosions and cysts may be seen.

Infection at the same site may give rise to a similar presentation but the red, tender skin is usually dry in gout while it feels wet in infection; the regional lymph nodes at the groin are usually tender and enlarged in the case of infection but not in gout. Local aspiration should only be attempted if there is a high suspicion of infection as the tenderness is usually extreme.

The acute attack is usually precipitated by a sudden rise in serum urate following excess alcohol, severe dieting or initiation of diuretic therapy. Surgery, severe systemic illness, trauma and unusual physical exercise may also precipitate an acute attack.

Secondary causes of gout should be excluded, e.g. diuretics, low doses of aspirin (less than 4 g), lymphomas, leukaemia, renal failure, excessive alcohol intake and severe widespread psoriasis.

The patient should be prescribed indomethacin, starting with a dose of 50–100 mg every 4 to 6 hours until the inflammation subsides; the dose can then be lowered to 25 mg t.d.s. for at least a month. If there is recurrence, the patient should go back to the higher dose. Colchicine is an alternative treatment, starting with 1 mg and then 0.5 mg every 2 to 3 hours until the pain is relieved or vomiting or diarrhoea occurs, or a total dose of 10 mg been taken. The maintenance dose is 0.5 mg three times a day.

Allopurinol, which inhibits xanthine oxidase hence preventing the conversion of xanthine and hypoxanthine to uric acid, is indicated if there are (1) tophi, (2) repeated attacks and (3) associated uric acid renal calculi. It should be given from 3 to 6 months after the acute attack has subsided and with a covering dose of indomethacin (25 mg t.d.s.) or colchicine (0.5 mg t.d.s.) as it may itself precipitate an acute attack for a further 3 months. The allopurinol therapy should be life-long.

INFLAMMATORY ARTHRITIS

The feet are involved in 90% of cases of rheumatoid arthritis. Commonly it is the MTP joints which are the first to be involved symmetrically with swelling and tenderness. Continued inflammation of the MTP, subtaloid and other small joints leads to laxity of the supporting tissues causing the late deformities of the rheumatoid foot: loss of the longitudinal arch (pes planus), hallux valgus, hammer toes, fibular deviation of the toes, valgus deformity of the hindfoot and subluxation of the MTP joints with painful callosities underneath.

Regular chiropody is needed. Many patients need well-padded surgical shoes with arch-supporting insoles as well as metatarsal supports. Severe valgus deformity of the hindfoot may require a below-knee orthosis consisting of a single outside iron bar with a T-strap. Severe cases may require triple arthrodesis and an MTP arthroplasty (Fowler's operation) with very good results.

Psoriasis, Reiter's syndrome and the colitic arthropathies may also affect the feet. The involvement of the joints is usually asymmetrical, and in a case of psoriasis there are usually nail changes. The involved toes may look swollen and red with extreme tenderness due to involvement of the joints as well as the tendons (hence the term 'sausage toe').

MARCH FRACTURE (STRESS FRACTURE)

This commonly occurs at the back of the second or third metatarsal bone. There is often a history of prolonged unaccustomed walking. A slight swelling may be visible at the base of the affected metatarsal accompanied by local tenderness on wriggling the same bone. The X-ray often shows a hairline crack or callous formation but may be negative: in the latter case a radioisotope scan is usually positive.

For a rapid recovery the foot should be put in a walking POP cast or Baycast for 6 weeks.

DIFFUSE FOOT PAIN

There should be no difficulty in diagnosing the ischaemic, diabetic or neuropathic foot if proper physical examination and urine examination are conducted routinely. When diabetes mellitus is diagnosed, the patient should be given clear instructions (verbal or in the form of a leaflet) on how to look after his feet regularly and properly; this prevents many later complications.

Table 11.4 *Causes of diffuse foot pain*

Peripheral vascular disease
Diabetic Charcot's joint
Tarsal tunnel syndrome (compression of posterior tibial nerve)
Sudeck's atrophy
Peripheral neuropathy (diabetic or otherwise)

12

Rehabilitation of Patients with Rheumatic Diseases

□ □ □ □ □ □ □ □ □ □ □ □ □

The aim of successful rehabilitation of patients with rheumatic diseases is restoration to full employment and social participation. However, this is not always possible in severely affected arthritic patients and the elderly, where achievement of independence in self-care may be equally important.

The pattern of care of arthritic patients involves five main aims:

(1) Pain relief.
(2) Prevention of deformity.
(3) Correction of existing deformity.
(4) Improvement in functional and vocational capabilities.
(5) Halting the disease process if at all possible.

To achieve these aims, proper medical management with judicious and timely surgical intervention is needed, supported by physiotherapy, occupational therapy and nursing care. In addition, valuable contributions can be made by the social worker, the local ALAC (Artificial Limb and Appliance Centre) medical officer, the chiropodist, the disablement resettlement officer and the psychologist. Because of the chronic nature of most rheumatic diseases, the patient has to be seen regularly by his general practitioner, hospital doctor and the above paramedical disciplines. The patient needs to be educated about the disease and given adequate explanation of its history, and the patient's own role in influencing the progress of the disease should also be stressed. The Arthritis and Rheumatism Council booklets on rheumatoid arthritis, osteoarthritis, neck pain, gout, ankylosing spondylitis, lumbar disc disorders, etc. are very helpful in achieving the latter. The patient should also be instructed to try and maintain a balance between rest and activity and to try to rearrange his lifestyle in such a way as to avoid fatigue and pain whenever possible.

Table 12.1 *General assessment of the arthritic patient*

Clinical, laboratory and radiological assessment
Activities of daily living
Mobility (indoor and outdoor)
Home and social situation
Finance
Work
Recreation and hobbies
Psychological status

THE ROLE OF THE GENERAL PRACTITIONER

The family doctor can act as the co-ordinator of the community services the patient needs. He is capable of treating most patients with osteoarthritis and soft tissue lesions as well as some of the patients with rheumatoid arthritis, especially when he has access to a physiotherapy service and the services of an occupational therapist. Gold and penicillamine therapy can be supervised by the family doctor.

Table 12.2 *Community services*

Home help
Community nurse
Community physiotherapist
Health visitor
Rehabilitation officer (community occupational therapist)
Chiropodist
Over 60's club
'Meals on wheels'
Voluntary services
Social Services department
DHSS allowances

THE ROLE OF THE PHYSIOTHERAPIST

In the acute phase the affected joint should be rested, and if there are several joints affected then bed rest should be prescribed with adequate splinting of the affected joints to avoid deformities. When the acute phase has subsided, the physiotherapist starts to mobilize the patient and teaches him a set of exercises which he must do regularly to maintain the maximum range of movements in his joints and to avoid deformity.

The patient's compliance with home exercise may be greater if he has to return regularly for assessment. For those arthritic patients who would require ambulance transport to attend the hospital outpatient physiotherapy department, it is much cheaper and more convenient to use the community physiotherapy service.

THE ROLE OF THE OCCUPATIONAL THERAPIST

The contribution of the occupational therapist is invaluable in assessing the patient's degree of independence, personal care, mobility, dexterity, his home situation and his hobbies and outdoor activities. If the patient is disabled, a home visit would be helpful to find out the patient's difficulties and correct them accordingly. These home visits may have to be repeated every 6–12 months or earlier if the deterioration is quicker. There are many aids and appliances which are helpful in maintaining the patient's independence (see Table 12.3).

Table 12.3 *Some practical aids to the arthritic patient*

Home care	Large-handled door key, grip mats, long-handled dustpan and brush, retrieving sticks, trolleys, electric plug with handle, footmops.
Kitchen	Adapted cutlery, wire basket, pegboards, milk bottle holders.
Bathroom	'Grip kit', soap holder, flush panels, bath steps, bath boards, long-handled washers, thermostatic shower.
Toilet	Raised toilet seats, commodes.
Hoists	Electric or hydraulic.
Dressing and grooming	Velcro (instead of buttons), elastic shoelaces, stocking aids, dressing stick, long-handled comb, long-handled shoe horn.
Wheelchairs	Self-propelled, attendant-propelled, power-propelled.
Gardening	Long-handled utensils, soil miller, kneeler stool, hose control.
Driving	Rotating (swivelling) car seats, throttle pedal, switch extensions.

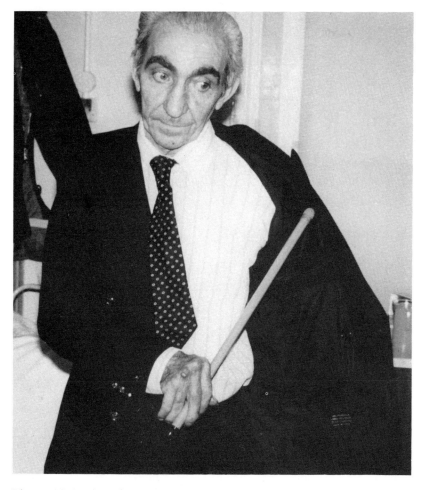

Figure 12.1 A patient with severe rheumatoid arthritis undressing with the help of a stick supplied by the Occupational Therapist.

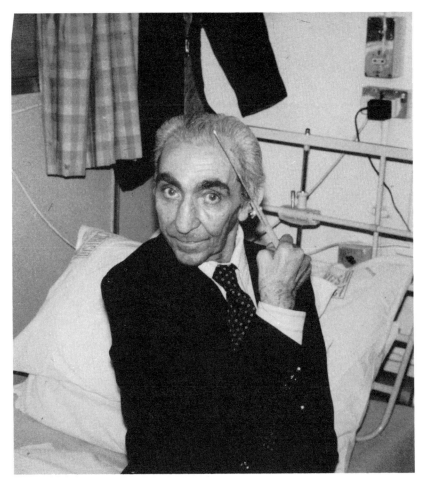

Figure 12.2 A comb with a long handle will help a patient with severe
rheumatoid arthritis to comb his hair.

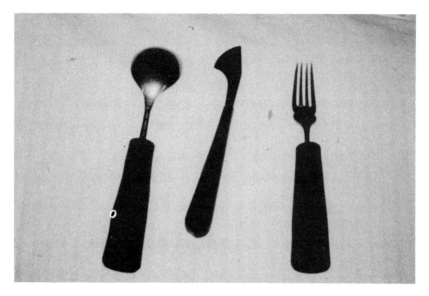

Figure 12.3   Special cutlery for a patient with rheumatoid arthritis.

WHEELCHAIRS

The severely disabled arthritic will find that a wheelchair increases his mobility and his independence (see Table 12.4). If he has a companion who is able-bodied, a pushchair can be very useful: Model 9 can be folded and carried in most car boots and Model 10 fits into a Mini. Model 8 would be suitable if the patient can wheel himself. Powered wheelchairs are rarely supplied by the DHSS for outdoor use, and the patient may have to buy one privately. The patient with rheumatoid arthritis whose mobility has suffered may be given a powered wheelchair sooner to prevent any deterioration in the function of the joints of the upper limbs.

Table 12.4 *Examples of the wheelchairs supplied by the Department of Health and Social Security*

---

(1) Occupant-controlled wheelchairs suitable for indoor and outdoor use, and can be folded:
   Model 7 (can be carried even in small cars)
   Model 8 (can be carried in most cars)

(2) Pushchairs – lightweight folding car chairs mainly for outdoor use:
   Model 9
   Model 10 (can be carried even in small cars)

(3) Occupant-controlled powered chairs – for indoor use only, cannot be folded:
   Model 109 (modified 9L), better than the AC Epic 102 chair
   Model 103 is shorter

For the full range of wheelchairs consult the DHSS Handbook of Wheelchairs, Bicycles and Tricycles

---

WORK AND TRANSPORT

If the patient is working, the treating doctor has to determine whether the patient is able to go back to his previous job, or whether he may need to change it. The Disablement Resettlement Officer (DRO) is usually able to advise and help with this: the majority of DRO's work from employment offices or job centres, but a small number are based in hospitals. Sometimes the patient may be able to do his job but because of his severe stiffness and disability he is unable to get up from bed, change his clothes and then travel the long journey to his place of work. The problem is compounded if he is unable to drive. This is why an arthritic patient who is able to drive should be encouraged to continue to do so, but may need some aids or modification to the car, e.g. a wide-angled rear view mirror, a good head rest, swivelling seats, special seats to avoid backache, switch extensions, extra large control knobs or even automatic transmission

The patient who is unable to walk or virtually unable to walk and is between 5 and 65 years old, would qualify for mobility allowance (MA) (£20 in 1984) which is non-taxable. It can be used to buy a car or an outdoor powered wheelchair via a charity (Motability) through a hire purchase scheme. All mobility allowance beneficiaries qualify for exemption from vehicle excise duty. Once granted, MA continues to be paid until the patient is 75 years old.

Table 12.5 *Allowances and Benefits for which a disabled person may be eligible*

Sickness Benefit	One adult dependent; less for each dependent child.
Invalidity Benefit	Usually replaces Sickness Benefit after 168 days (or 120 days in certain circumstances) of entitlement.
Unemployment Benefit	Limited in duration to 312 days in any one period of interruption of employment.
Attendance Allowance (AA)	Tax-free allowance for severely disabled people including children over the age of 2 years. There are two rates.
Invalid Car Allowance	Payable to men and single women of working age who are unable to work because of the need to stay at home and care for severely disabled person in receipt of AA or constant AA.
Non-contributory Invalidity Pension	Not dependent on contributions and might be payable if the claimant does not qualify for contributory benefit.
Mobility Allowance	Non-taxable, available to people between 5 and 65 who are unable or virtually unable to walk because of physical disability.
Disablement Allowance	Newly introduced.
Disablement Benefit	Usually paid 15 weeks after an industrial accident or onset of disease.
Family Income Supplement	Payable to families with low incomes where head of family is in full-time paid work and there is at least one dependent child in the family.
Supplementary Benefit	Payable if beneficiary does not have to satisfy any contribution condition.

INDIVIDUAL JOINTS

Patients with rheumatoid arthritis need to be reviewed every 6–12 months on average in a combined rheumatological–orthopaedic clinic in the presence of a rheumatologist and an orthopaedic surgeon who are experienced in rheumatoid disease and its complications.

Maintenance of optimal body weight is important. The work load on a weight-bearing joint is about five times the body weight; a reduction of 1 kg leads to a 5 kg load reduction on the knee or hip on weight bearing. If this factor of five is explained to the obese patient, he will probably be more enthusiastic about body weight reduction.

The knee and hip joints only are described below as most other joints have been dealt with in other chapters (see Chapters 7, 8, 9 and 11 on the back, neck, shoulder and foot, respectively).

The knee joint

Aspiration of knee effusion followed by immobilization of the leg in POP back slab for a few days leads to rapid relief of pain. An effusion in the knee causes a reciprocal inhibition and later wasting of the quadriceps femoris muscle, therefore teaching the patient exercises to strengthen this muscle breaks the vicious circle which eventually makes the knee unstable. If there is synovitis an intra-articular steroid injection leads to rapid pain relief lasting for 3–6 weeks. Heat, ice, ultrasound and interferential therapy may help ease the pain for a while but the effect is rarely long-lasting. A walking stick used in the opposite hand may relieve 50% of the pressure on the affected knee if used properly: the stick should be of the proper length (from greater trochanter to the floor) and must have a ferrule at the end. If the patient's hand is deformed a special moulded handle may be used.

Flexion contractures may be prevented by night splinting and, if they are already established, gradual stretching using repeated POP casts replaced every 5 days may lead to knee strengthening.

Moderate valgus or varus deformity pain on walking may be relieved with a lightweight telescopic valgus support (TVS brace). Unstable knees which eventually require replacement may be made more stable using a knee cage or a full length lightweight caliper known as KAFO (Knee Ankle Foot Orthosis) The patient who suffers pain on going down stairs (usually caused by patello-femoral disease) may find relief on descending backwards.

Medical (using radioactive yttrium-90) or surgical synovectomy may be indicated in persistent knee synovitis. Unstable, deformed knees causing pain on resting, at night and on walking require a knee replacement, but the results are not as good as for hip replacement.

The hip joint

Flexion contracture of the hip may be prevented by regular periods of prone lying for at least half an hour a day. As with the knee, a walking stick in the contralateral hand is useful. Exercises to strengthen the hip muscles are useful and may be more effective if done in a hydrotherapy pool. Other forms of physiotherapy may also give palliative relief. If the damaged joints are causing severe pain during the night and on weight bearing, then total hip replacement is indicated: the results are good.

13

Drugs in Rheumatology

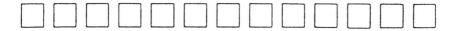

INTRODUCTION

The drugs available in rheumatology can be divided into three main groups:

(1)   The analgesics.
(2)   The non-steroidal anti-inflammatory drugs.
(3)   Disease modifying antirheumatic drugs.

Table 13.1 *Analgesics*

Aspirin (low dose)

Paracetamol

Paracetamol combinations including benorylate and Distalgesic

Codeine, dihydrocodeine (DF118), Fortral, mefenamic acid, flufenamic acid

---

Table 13.2 *Non-steroidal anti-inflammatory drugs (NSAIDs)*

---

1. *Drugs with short half life*
    Aspirin (3.6 g per day or more)
    Indomethacin
    Proprionic acid derivates including ibuprofen, ketoprofen, naproxen, diclofenac, tiaprofenic acid
    Azapropazone

2. *Longer acting drugs*
    Fenbufen, piroxicam, Isoxicam

3. *Slow release preparations*
    Keoprofen, Voltarol slow release, Indocid-R

4. *Drugs available as suppositories*
    Indomethacin, sulindac, tiaprofenic acid, naproxen, ketoprofen

5. *Drugs withdrawn*
    Benoxaprofen, phenylbutazone and its derivatives, Osmosin, indoprofen

---

Table 13.3 *Disease modifying antirheumatic drugs (DMARDs)*

Antimalarials (chloroquine), gold, penicillamine

Immunosuppressive drugs
Azathioprine, cyclophosphamide, methotrexate, chlorambucil

Drugs for which claims have been made
Fenclofenac, Alclofenac, Salazopyrin, thympoietin

There is a bewildering number of drugs available to treat patients suffering from rheumatic diseases and their associated problems: in this chapter the idea is to give guidelines where possible. Simple analgesics have a role in the treatment of pain, primarily in the absence of inflammation. This is suitable treatment for the majority of patients with osteoarthritis who will benefit from a drug such as a low dose aspirin (2 g daily) or paracetamol (up to 3 g daily) in one or other of its combination forms. It is also appropriate for short-term pain as in the majority of patients who suffer from backache or neck pain. Inflammatory disease requires anti-inflammatory therapy; however, no anti-inflammatory drug given in adequate dosage is free of the problems of gastrointestinal irritation. The non-steroidal with the lowest gastrointestinal irritant profile at the moment appears to be Lederfen. The reason why so many drugs have appeared in this area is that the side effects profile for each new one is superior to aspirin. In all probability, the reason for this superiority has been less efficacy due to lower dosage. Few trials have been carried out against aspirin; these are difficult to carry out because of the specific side effects which aspirin induces, leading to the removal of 'blindness'".

We would recommend strongly the use of aspirin for the treatment of acute rheumatoid arthritis and acute painful inflammatory joints. It is necessary to give enough in order to obtain the necessary effect; this involves 4 g a day at least, preferably in divided doses 4 times a day. Enteric-coated aspirin has the same effect as aspirin with a slight lessening of the side effects. Trilisate (choline magnesium trisalicylate) is available but in our experience the incidence of side effects is similar to that observed with sodium salicylate. Often it is necessary to combine aspirin with a non-steroidal anti-inflammatory drug such as indomethacin (75 mg at night) or naproxen (500 mg at night) to relieve morning stiffness connected with the inflammatory disease.

GASTROINTESTINAL SIDE EFFECTS

If the patient develops indigestion, there is an argument for trying another non-steroidal anti-inflammatory drug. Side effects tend to be idiosyncratic: a patient who develops side effects on one drug may well not develop them on another. Unfortunately side effects can occur at any time, although studies we have carried out show that they tend to occur either very early in the course of treatment, or at around 3 months with NSAIDs. If a patient develops peptic ulceration there is a strong argument for stopping the NSAIDs. Any patient with persistent indigestion should be subject to barium studies and gastroscopy to exclude underlying peptic ulceration. In patients with existing abdominal pain, it may be worth a trial of a suppository formulation in order to avoid local causes of irritation; however, the systemic effect of NSAIDs is just as important in the role of causing ulcers as local effects, and suppositories do not always achieve the desired effect. They are also unpleasant to use, particularly for patients with rheumatoid arthritis who may have difficulty in insertion. There is a further problem today in that generic suppositories may crumble: we have seen this with generic indomethacin suppositories and there is an argument for using brand names in this situation.

EXTRA DRUGS TO TREAT ARTHRITIS

Depression is sometimes a major feature in the patient suffering from arthritis, and antidepressants such as amitriptyline or nortrip-tyline, particularly given at night, may achieve more than either increasing the anti-inflammatory medication, or using disease modifying antirheumatic therapy. For backache, simple analgesics may not be enough to relieve the patient's suffering which is often due to severe muscle spasm and may be best relieved by large doses of diazepam (Valium); up to 25 mg daily may be necessary to relax the patient for muscle spasm to settle down. There is no place in the treatment of rheumatic diseases for the use of opiates and narcotic medications: these are to be strongly resisted.

FURTHER TREATMENT OF RHEUMATOID ARTHRITIS

If the use of non-steroidal anti-inflammatory drugs fails and the patient's disease continues to remain active, there is an argument for the use of either gold (Myocrisin) or penicillamine. Some GPs are perfectly able to make the decision as to the need for these drugs and the monitoring required when they are used on a regular basis. However, the majority of general practitioners prefer to send the patient to the hospital outpatients department where this decision can be made. The patient can be monitored regularly, the management then being combined between the hospital consultant and the general practitioner.

Injections of Myocrisin (50 mg) are required to be given weekly after an initial 10 mg test dose. Monitoring of the full blood count plus platelets should be carried out every 2 weeks up to 8 weeks, then monthly *indefinitely* thereafter. Urine testing can be done either by the clinic nurse or better still, by the patient himself. It is easy to teach patients to use dipsticks. Patients should also be warned of the possibility of itching and skin rash which can develop on treatment with both gold and penicillamine. Other side effects encountered with penicillamine include myasthenia gravis, occasionally lupus syndromes, late rashes and loss of taste in 10% of patients treated. Sometimes these side effects are severe enough to lead to the withdrawal of the drug; again these decisions are perhaps better made in a hospital environment. Immunosuppressives should be reserved for patients in whom gold or penicillamine has failed to produce the desired effect. Amyloidosis, a complication of rheumatoid arthritis or psoriatic arthropathy, is occasionally remedied by the use of chlorambucil but this is not a particularly successful form of medication in the adult.

THE USE OF STEROIDS

Steroids should not be used on a regular basis for the treatment of rheumatoid arthritis and never for osteoarthritis. There are, however, exceptional instances where they may be used by hospital consultants in conjunction with the general practitioner. Polymyalgia rheumatica and temporal arteritis are specific indications for corticosteroids: prednisolone is often used with a dose of 40 mg for the latter condition, and 20 mg for the former. Patients then have to be weaned off this medication using the ESR and the clinical symptomatology as the guidelines.

Systemic lupus erythematosus, when it involves renal lesions or cerebral lesions, may well require the use of corticosteroids, probably along with immunosuppressive drugs in order to keep the dosage as low as possible. The vexed question of the treatment of rheumatoid arthritis with steroids is still hotly controversial. Alternate daily steroids are useful for children with Still's disease, as given this way the growth spurt is no longer suppressed to the degree that it is if the steroids are given daily. In the adult, steroids should really only be used in *life-threatening circumstances* where the patient's life expectancy is less than the time taken to develop side effects, e.g. patients with very severe stiffness in the elderly age group where 5–10 mg last thing at night may be extremely helpful. Recently, there has been popular use of soluble methyl-prednisolone 1 g infusion. This is of use for severe rheumatoid arthritis and is a means of 'buying' three months at the most, thus enabling the patient to start taking a disease modifying drug such as gold or penicillamine and to have relief of symptoms until the drug begins to work. This is not suitable for all patients: it is to be avoided in patients with peptic ulceration, but is nevertheless symptomatically useful for patients with severe rheumatic disease. It has the advantage over oral prednisolone of being non-addictive, as treatment is in the form of a 'one-off' injection.

FURTHER RESEARCH

Whilst many new non-steroidal drugs are being developed, these provide only symptomatic remedy, i.e. relief of pain and symptoms but not suppression of the disease itself. There is continuing research into the use of disease modifying antirheumatic drugs, but it is difficult to find drugs which are non-toxic. The ideal anti-rheumatic therapy has still not been found which is why so many alternatives exist. The use of superoxide radical scavengers is being evaluated in OA and RA. So far NSAIDs have been developed which block only the cyclo-oxygenase pathway: the research continues with agents able to block the alternative (lipo-oxygenase) pathway. The aim of these agents is to give the advantages of steroids without side effects.

14

Alternative Medicine

□ □ □ □ □ □ □ □ □ □ □ □

Most general practitioners are now subject to patients coming along and demanding alternative medicine. The usual complaint is that the patient has suffered from ordinary conventional medicine and has gained no benefit from it. They may have attended a hospital, may have been prescribed drugs and developed side effects, or maybe their condition has just not altered and they are in a desperate situation.

The problem with most alternative medical techniques is that they have not been submitted to the rigours of a true clinical study to determine their merits or otherwise. We at King's College Hospital have tried very hard to submit some of the alternative techniques which are available to such trials, and in many cases we have found them to be wanting. In this chapter we have attempted to define the areas where alternative medicine is available, and to offer some hopefully balanced but inevitably personal attitudes towards their usefulness or otherwise. In part, alternative medicine has had a good press: firstly this is due to newspapers where articles commonly appear telling the public of its merits, and secondly the perpetrators of alternative medicine are allowed to advertise as they are not offering conventional medicine. Schools exist to teach people homoeopathy and osteopathy, but unfortunately a large number of practitioners has sprung up often without qualifications or training from whom there is no protection for the public. Dangers are possible for the unwary, therefore it is wrong for patients to visit an alternative medicine practitioner unless recommended by a general practitioner or a consultant specialist: there should be an honest regard for scientific attainment.

The placebo effect is very strong in medicine. There is no doubt of its relevance to conventional medicine and in many clinical trials placebo is demonstrated as being a highly effective remedy. There is also no doubt that there is a placebo effect in alternative medicine, but the open question is whether any alternative medicine offers more than the simple placebo.

ACUPUNCTURE

Acupuncture has a long established historical background, being the treatment of choice for many medical ailments as performed in China. So effective is it in that country that it is even used for major abdominal surgery in preference to anaesthesia. A large number of theories have been advanced as to why it is effective, if indeed it is. The theory most acceptable to modern medical practice is that the insertion of needles into points leads to the release of central mediated chemicals (endorphins) which are actually able to control pain centrally. Unfortunately, the studies that have so far been published on the correlation between acupuncture and endorphin levels are slight: more work needs to be done to determine the relationship between these two things. One area of interest is the fact that needles put in one point can lead to pain relief whilst placed in other points the same relief is not achieved. Maybe there is more to it than endorphin release, and perhaps the Chinese mystic does provide some underlying answers.

We carried out a study where we compared acupuncture, conventional injection, anti-inflammatory drugs and physiotherapy along with placebo in the treatment of painful shoulder. We found all treatments to be equally effective. Perhaps this is a reflection of the fact that this condition would automatically get better anyway.

The risk from acupuncture is that potentially the needles can give rise to infection unless they are carefully sterilized; otherwise it would appear to be a procedure without risk. Perhaps the biggest risk is the practitioner who might use this treatment for wrong indication. Articles in the lay press have suggested that acupuncture can be used for cardiac failure or infection, and this is where the technique will develop a bad name. In the opinion of the authors, it is a technique which should be reserved for patients with intractable pain for whom conventional treatments have failed. If the patient then derives a temporary relief from his pain, the course of acupuncture will have been seen to have been a useful agent.

HOMOEOPATHY

The objective of homoeopathy is that patients can be treated with a substance which in one dilution can actually exacerbate symptoms, whereas in different dilution the patient's symptoms are relieved. The substances tend to be naturally occurring ones. Homoepathists like general physicians are concerned also with the whole patient, therefore in a homoeopathic appointment a patient is assessed not only for his medical condition, but also overall.

Studies

There is no doubt that a percentage of the population derives benefit from homoeopathic remedies. How much this is due to the remedy itself and how much the fact that somebody is taking an interest in the patient it is hard to be sure. A study was carried out between King's College Hospital, the Homoeopathic Hospital, Tonbridge and the Royal Homoeopathic Hospital, Queen's Square, London. Patients with osteoarthritis took part in a controlled 3-way double blind study between Rhustox (extract of poison ivy), placebo and a non-steroidal anti-inflammatory drug. All measurements were in favour of the non-steroidal anti-inflammatory drug, whether the patients were attending King's College Hospital or the homoepathic institutions. Of particular import was that patient preference was strongly in favour of the allopathic remedy. Homoeopathic comment on this study was that five patients receiving homoeopathic remedy actually had an exacerbation of their symptoms. These might have been the five patients who one would have expected to derive benefit from changing the dilution of the homoeopathic remedy. Our study was in all honesty a small tip of a large iceberg. We feel that much more research needs to be carried out in perhaps the same sort of way as we were able to work in order to assess the merits or otherwise of homoeopathy.

The danger is that people who purport to offer homoeopathic remedies may in fact put agents known to be highly effective but also toxic in the remedies. For example, we have come across the use of Russell's viper venom in low dilution known to be a very highly potent anti-inflammatory agent. This was being given to a patient without the patient being informed as to what he was receiving. In other countries there is the risk that a homoeopathic remedy may also include corticosteroids. Perhaps the best way around this is for the homoeopathists to work more closely in conjunction with their general physician colleagues: only in this way can respectability be maintained.

OSTEOPATHY

The idea of osteopathy, perhaps not far from reality, is that bones can be displaced. Certainly there is evidence that this can occur, for example in the cervical spine, and a lot of conventional physiotherapy is aimed at restoring normal posture. Where osteopathy becomes a little more difficult for conventional physicians to follow is in the area of instant cure. Again, no satisfactorily controlled studies of osteopathy have been carried out and the reason for this is perhaps the total conviction and confidence which the osteopaths have in what they do. In all probability, osteopathy in the right patient has an important role. The right patient is somebody who has been selected by the general practitioner or a consultant physician, for whom a full list of examination, history taking and investigations has been carried out and an accurate diagnosis has been made. If the diagnosis shows a mechanical problem as the cause of pain then osteopathy may well be a sensible line of treatment. The danger is that patients will refer themselves to non-medically qualified osteopaths and will end up with hemiplegia or paraplegia as a result of treatment carried out in the absence of an accurate diagnosis. This is why it is important that osteopaths work in conjunction with general physicians.

DIET

All sorts of diets have been suggested as having a role in the treatment of arthritis. The area of most interest is the Dong diet. Dr Dong, a Chinese physician, himself suffered from rheumatoid arthritis. He decided in his infinite wisdom that he should resort to the sort of food his mother used to give him. Living as he did in the poor areas of China, he lived on fish and a little rice, and wonder of wonders, his rheumatoid arthritis went away and never returned. Books appeared extolling the virtues of this diet, and many patients particularly in America swear by the Dong diet. Recently a study has been carried out to evaluate the Dong diet and to compare it with a controlled diet. The results were interesting in that there was no difference between the Dong and placebo diets in the treatment of arthritis, with the sole exception of two patients who when exposed to the Dong diet did make a miraculous recovery. Interestingly enough, when they were re-exposed to ordinary food their condition deteriorated. On taking away the ordinary food and re-introducing the Dong diet, the patients recovered again.

There may well be a small subgroup of patients who when treated with specialized diets may have an exacerbation of their joints. It is difficult to establish this particular group: there are people who assess hypersensitivity to various trace metals and other elements based on study of hair: how reliable this is is unclear at the moment. It seems logical to extend the work on diets to look in more detail at the question of whether diets are or are not meaningful. Certainly, in the view of the authors there is no harm in trying patients on exclusion diets should they so wish: on the other hand, they are not without their dangers. One patient recently at King's demanded to go on milk and honey: six weeks later she came back claiming a miraculous cure, but six weeks after that she came back with a severe rheumatoid exacerbation. Rheumatoid arthritis is a disease of relapses and remissions and therefore immediate response to a diet may well be a natural remission rather than anything whatsoever related to the diet.

OTHER REMEDIES

All sorts of other remedies are available to the general public from a herbalist's shop where they can buy devil's claw, Russell's viper venom or even extract of green limpet mussel. The last of these has been put to clinical trial and compared as if it were a non-steroidal anti-inflammatory drug, and it was shown to have no more effect than placebo. Maybe the ingestion of nasty smelling substances does have something like a placebo effect. All these unconventional remedies do need to be subject to clear tests and quality control. The anxiety of the authors is that in the absence of quality control and Committee on Safety of Medicines supervision, we have no idea how toxic these agents are. Extract of green limpet, for example, is a food and therefore has never been subject to a toxicity trial. As so many members of the general public have bought these remedies over the counter, one would like to see them registered as drugs at least from the point of view of proper evaluation.

Copper bracelets

Vast numbers of patients have faith in copper bracelets. A small study reported that some 6% of patients derived benefit from them, although there is no logical reason why copper bracelets should be effective in the treatment of arthritis. A more formal study as to their merits or otherwise would be appropriate. In all probability they are unlikely to cause much harm, unless copper itself may be absorbed.

CONCLUSION

Alternative medicine will continue to flourish whilst the general physicians who provide only primary care are not interested in this area. Some of the techniques probably have something to offer patients in individual situations, and it is up to the clinician to decide the correct indication for each of these procedures.

Appendix

□ □ □ □ □ □ □ □ □ □ □ □ □

Voluntary organizations in the UK

(Education, research, co-ordination, information, holidays, aids, etc.)

The British League against Rheumatism
c/o ARC, 41 Eagle Street, London WC1R 4AR
Tel. 01 405 8572

The Arthritis and Rheumatism Council for Research
41 Eagle Street, London WC1R 4AR
Tel. 01 405 8572

Arthritis Care (The British Rheumatism and Arthritis Association)
6 Grosvenor Crescent, London SW1X 7ER
Tel 01 235 0902

The Back Pain Association
31–33 Park Road, Teddington, Middlesex TW11 0AB
Tel. 01 977 1171

The Royal Association for Disability and Rehabilitation (RADAR)
25 Mortimer Street, London W1N 8AB
Tel. 01 637 5400

117

The Disabled Living Foundation
346 Kensington High Street, London W14 8NS
Tel. 01 602 2491

The Bath Institute of Rheumatic Diseases
Barton Meade House, Haydon, Radstock, Bath BA3 3QS
Tel. 0761 32472

The Leonard Cheshire Foundation
7 Market Mews, London W1Y 8HP
Tel 01 499 2665

The Horder Centre for Arthritics (Rehabilitation)
Crowborough, Sussex TN6 1XP
Tel. Crowborough 4141

The Committee on Sexual Problems for the Disabled (SPOD)
25 Mortimer Street, London W1N 8AB
Tel. 01 637 5400

Scottish Council on Disability
Princes House, 5 Shandwick Place, Edinburgh 2
Tel. 031 229 8632

The British Red Cross Society
9 Grosvenor Crescent, London SW1X 7EG
Tel. 01 235 5454

The Disabled Drivers' Association
Ashwellthorpe Hall, Ashwellthorpe, Norwich NR16 1EX
Tel. 050 841 449

The British Society of Motoring Disability Training Centre
102 Sydney Street, London SW3
Tel. 01 351 2377

Motability
The Adelphi, John Adam Street, London WC2N 6AZ
Tel. 01 839 5191

Queen Elizabeth Foundation for the Disabled
Leatherhead Court, Leatherhead, Surrey KT22 0BN
Tel. 01 970 2204

Banstead Place
Park Road, Banstead, Surrey SM7 3EE
Tel. 25 56222/51756
(Patient may try a range of powered wheelchairs and other transport vehicles designed for the disabled.)

Index

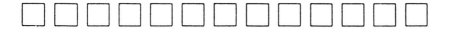